From Time to Eternity and Back

A Priest's Successful Struggle With Cancer

FATHER JOSEPH M. CHAMPLIN

Rector, Cathedral of the Immaculate Conception

ST PAULS

Alba House

Bottom right photo on front cover, copyright © 2002, Ron Trinca Photography.

Library of Congress Cataloging-in-Publication Data

Champlin, Joseph M.
  From time to eternity and back / Joseph M. Champlin.
    p. cm.
  ISBN 0-8189-0962-5
  1. Champlin, Joseph M. 2. Catholic Church—United
States—Clergy—Biography. 3. Cancer—Patients—United
States—Biography. I. Title

  BX4705.C447A3 2003
  282'.092—dc22

                      2003019369

Imprimatur:
✠ Most Reverend Thomas J. Costello, DD
Vicar General, Diocese of Syracuse, New York
Exaltation of the Holy Cross
September 14, 2003

Produced and designed in the United States of America by the
Fathers and Brothers of the Society of St. Paul,
2187 Victory Boulevard, Staten Island, New York 10314-6603,
as part of their communications apostolate.

ISBN: 0-8189-0962-5

Printing Information:

Current Printing - first digit	1	2	3	4	5	6	7	8	9	10

Year of Current Printing - first year shown

2004	2005	2006	2007	2008	2009	2010	2011	2012

Table of Contents

Introduction vii

Part I: Struggling with Cancer

1. Surprise 3
2. Shadow on the Horizon 5
3. A Dark Cloud Descends 9
4. Waiting 13
5. Bad News/Good News 17
6. Public Disclosure 21
7. A Sick Puppy 32
8. Absorbed 39
9. Eternal Life and Temporary Conversions 43
10. The Healing Process Continues 51
11. An Incredible Wave of Support 58
12. Reviewing One's Life 65
13. How Do You Feel? 71
14. The Road To Recovery 74

Part II: One Year Later

15. An Incredibly Successful Journey 89
16. Several Serious Scares and Divine Nudges 100
17. Looking Back and Ahead 108

Acknowledgments 115

Introduction

On a wintry February 2, 1956 at the Cathedral of the Immaculate Conception in Syracuse, New York I was ordained a Roman Catholic priest.

Nearly a half-century later, on another stormy February day, and after more than 70 years of practically perfect health, my life changed dramatically.

An oncologist determined and declared that I had Waldenstrom's Macroglobinemia, a rare form of bone marrow cancer.

These pages cover my struggles with this cancer from 2000-2003. They will sketch events prior to the final diagnosis, detail my life during the difficult, year-long treatment and describe the perhaps only temporary, but still quite incredible positive results from chemotherapy — full restoration of my health.

I wrote Part I, "Struggling With Cancer," while actively undergoing the first months of treatment. That section is, therefore, rather intense and highly personal.

I wrote Part II, as indicated, "One Year Later." It contains reflections upon the second half treatments, descriptions about the recovery of my health and observations concerning the future. That section is, consequently, less intense and more general.

I hope and I pray that this little book will be of some help to persons struggling with cancer and also to those who care for and about individuals afflicted with the disease.

Part I
Struggling with Cancer

Surprise

*E*arly on a May evening I left my center city Cathedral residence and drove out into the suburbs for a dinner engagement. I was to meet there a friend of more than fifty years for our regular meal and visit.

This is a routine for us: at the end of a previous dinner we check our schedules and reserve for another such session a night four to six weeks in the future. On those usually Sunday nights we enjoy the food, catch up on each other's lives and discuss matters of mutual interest.

Tonight's dinner and exchange would be a bit special. My birthday occurs around that time and he wanted to pick up the tab; I reciprocate on his in December.

Reaching the restaurant, I was puzzled to see him standing in the parking lot studying an appointment book. Normally, the first to arrive checks in, is seated and waits for the other. However, we simply exchanged greetings in the lot and as we walked into the restaurant I was clutching a file and some papers for later discussion.

When we made our way into the dining area, I noticed a couple of balloons and commented that it must be a special occasion for someone.

Then the lights went up, seventy people shouted "Happy

Birthday" and the celebration began, much to my absolutely total surprise. It is not easy to keep matters like these from me, but I had no inkling, not a clue or suspicion about this party.

My brother and his wife were there from Los Angeles, as well as my sister and her husband from New York City. Friends and colleagues from the past and the present made up the rest of the participants.

There were smiles and laughter as they observed the obviously dumbfounded priest whose 70th birthday had passed a few days earlier. Hugs and kisses, food and drink, toasts and roasts, cards and gifts, prayers and good wishes filled the next two hours.

Later I realized how delicate and difficult was the committee's task to bring about that surprise event.

I drove home alone or, rather, almost floated back to the Cathedral quite overwhelmed by this unexpected outpouring of love.

For years I have tried to spend a couple of hours at quiet prayer in the early morning. Following that pattern the next day, I silently reflected with a warm and grateful heart on the wonderful evening. But I also posed some questions to myself:

Seven decades of my life, of my time on earth have passed. What does the next decade hold?

Will I be alive ten years from now or will I have passed from here to eternity?

Where will I be living?

How many of those friends and colleagues will still be alive?

What will I be doing?

The questions, of course, were unanswerable. Partial responses to some of them would come soon enough.

Shadow on the Horizon

*P*laying sports and regularly exercising have been part of my life from the earliest days. For the initial dozen years in Hammondsport, New York, I would daily spend hours swimming in clear, beautiful Keuka Lake and often join in a pick-up softball game on the empty lot near my house and across from the Catholic Church.

I distinctly recall one day lofting a high foul fly ball which drifted through trees and crashed into the window of a house by the lot. We all of course, immediately scattered. My single parent mother subsequently insisted that I walk over to this house, apologize to its widow owner and offer to pay for the necessary repairs.

In my teens I played soccer, basketball and baseball during the school year. Summer meant catching for the local "town" baseball team on weekends. During the week I worked first as a farm laborer for a neighbor and later as a section hand on the railroad which passed through our area. Each night, however, I would pedal my bike a mile or so down the road to an abandoned sand mine operation whose clean, but cloudy waters gave me a chance for a long swim.

At the University of Notre Dame, I learned the wonderful Irish game of handball and for the next fifty years played several times a week until my regular partners were no longer available.

After ordination in 1956, I added basketball scrimmages with the high school team to the handball and swimming. But they soon proved to be too big, aggressive and fast for me. A broken nose from a flying elbow helped accelerate my decision to abandon active participation in that sport.

While pastor of Holy Family Church in Fulton, my barber, a veteran marathoner and erstwhile runner, suggested I try jogging. I half-heartedly worked at it during the winter months. However, six months later, on a June afternoon, I recall returning to the rectory and exclaiming to myself, "I just ran five miles."

Jogging for 4-6 miles now became an alternative to the handball and swimming. Since I also traveled extensively for lectures, running also gave me an opportunity to explore many locations here and abroad. That included Hawaii around Diamond Head, along the Panama Canal, South Africa, Rome and Italy, plus numerous places in Canada and throughout the United States.

Around my fiftieth birthday, I became owner of a cottage on Skaneateles Lake, a Finger Lake very similar to that body of water which was the site of my early swimming days. Because of its proximity to my work place, I now could easily drive out often for a long-distance, late afternoon swim.

When I was in my fifties my physician, an avid advocate of running and marathons, encouraged me to run one of those 26.2 mile races. I reluctantly agreed, trained strenuously for eight weeks and finished the Ottawa Marathon in a little less than four hours.

I never have run another one, but the Canadian experience taught me this valuable personal lesson. "Getting an hour of exercise five days a week is for me extremely beneficial — spiritually and emotionally, mentally and physically." Like many of my ideals and resolutions, I don't keep this goal perfectly. Either by jogging, occasional handball or long-distance swimming, I probably squeeze in that hour only two or three days weekly. But I remained convinced of its value for me.

A decade ago, I began to combine jogging for fun with running for funds.

Every Memorial Day the Town of Camillus sponsors its well-attended parade preceded by a 5K, 3.2 mile race. Following the example of some running friends and as pastor of the church in that town, I invited people to sponsor me in the race for $5. If I finished under 30 minutes, the money would go to D.A.R.E., an effort to counteract drug abuse in the community. With little promotion, over 50 people still supported my run and I thus raised some $300 for that good cause.

A few years later I became rector of the Cathedral in Syracuse and now had a new cause. This would be to support the over 100 boys and girls of our school, who are totally bi-racial and mostly not Catholic, with 75% from below poverty level households. We soon added another incentive: Contribution of $75 would entitle donors to "Dinner for Two" at a fine local restaurant.

The Camillus event became a very popular and successful undertaking. For example, the Memorial Day 2001 race attracted 469 donors who contributed $28,629 for our poor kids with 273 receiving Gift Certificates for Two.

However, at the race a shadow appeared on the horizon for me, an ominous warning that after all those years of fine health and of seemingly unlimited energy, something was happening to my body. For the first time in 30 years of running, I had to stop twice during that relatively brief race because of rather significant fatigue and shortness of breath. Moreover, I simply did not have the push to pick up my pace for the last 100 yards or so at the finish.

Two friends who greeted me at the end said I looked quite peaked and had dried salt around my mouth. Afterwards, at my cottage, I felt exhausted and dropped off into an unusually long nap.

For the decade previous to this, Dr. Gary Tyndall had become my personal physician and very close friend. Thinking my heart was complaining after the seven decades of vigorous exercise, I spoke to him about the experiences.

He arranged a stress test with a local cardiologist. Afterwards, the specialist commented: "Your heart is terrific for a man your age. No problem here." So that was not the cause of the difficulty.

The race phenomenon remained a puzzle. We finally attributed the experience to dehydration and forgot about it.

However, we later recalled that in another earlier context, my blood test had revealed a slight rise in an item used to measure the presence of a certain disease within the bone marrow. The increment was minimal and could be caused by a fluke in the test itself. We, too, dismissed that minor variation as insignificant.

Soon enough we came to realize, in retrospect, that the race itself and blood test result were slight shadows on my health horizon, shadows which would, in a few months, give way to a very dark cloud.

A Dark Cloud Descends

*I*nstant and uninterrupted sleep has been an enormous blessing for me. Whether at night or a nap, I fall asleep within record time after my head hits the pillow.

Up until recently, I have usually managed on about six hours sleep nightly, but always with a ten minute power nap every afternoon following a light lunch. In fact, without that brief mid-day break, the rest of the day becomes a strain for me.

Several years ago one of our custodians with whom I had worked closely for over a decade commented to me: "Some people who love you a lot think you need more rest."

They were right. A few telltale signs of sleep deprivation swiftly came into my mind.

After a lengthy dinner with friends, if there is a lull in the conversation, my eyes begin to droop. As I preside at late Sunday morning Masses while another preaches, I often have to fight drowsiness soon after the homily begins, much to the amusement of worshipers in the pews. One Saturday afternoon, following several weddings on a warm day, I sat down in the Reconciliation Room to hear confessions. Fatigue quickly took over. At one point, a voice on the other side of the divider asked: "Father, is it all right if I leave now?" Stunned out of my slumber, I was too chagrined to ask how long the person had been waiting to be dismissed.

All of this I attributed to my seventy years and began to expand both the six hours at night and the ten minutes in the afternoon.

However, some months after the Memorial Day race incident, a deeper kind of persistent weariness invaded my life. The naps grew longer and less refreshing. A receptionist recalls my remark: "I just had a long nap, yet I still feel tired and without energy."

About that time, in October, I developed a hard and ugly, yet dry cough. There was no expectoration, but the cough was both distressing and debilitating to me and surely disturbing to parishioners. "Will he make it through the homily and the Mass?", I imagined them saying to themselves and to one another.

My personal physician tried everything both to determine the cause of the cough and a cure for it. But the cough continued with sustained vehemence, exacerbated right after Christmas by a bout with the flu.

Around the holidays, the physician ordered another blood test, including a sample of that particular item which had surfaced at a 350 count about one year earlier. To our dismay, the number had now zoomed to an alarming 1500 in a relatively few months.

Dr. Tyndall telephoned a local oncologist who said the rapid increment was significant, but that they normally do not become concerned until the figure reaches 3000. Nevertheless, he agreed to see me in a few weeks prior to my departure for ten days of vacation in a warmer climate.

During this period, I had cut back on my running because of the continuing fatigue and the shortness of breath. Moreover, I was having some distress in my right knee.

I called Dr. John Fatti, an orthopedic specialist and long-time friend, who brought me into his office and did an X-ray on the knee. "Father, you have great knees for a man your age. I see nothing unusual."

His remark brought back a comment made to me some time before while I was jogging in a troubled area of our city. I passed by a woman, apparently of ill repute, who turned and commented, "Great legs."

This was surely an affirming comment for an older man, even though the source of the praise raises some question about its authenticity.

Dr. John suggested I cold wrap the knee at night and take an anti-inflammatory pill each day. The soreness soon disappeared and I learned that a packet of frozen peas and carrots works better than ice cubes in treating a knee. They more successfully mold to the knee and leg.

To my surprise, four days later the knee began to swell considerably. Dr. Fatti, who in connection with my physician knew about the blood development and was concerned about the persistent cough, then ordered an MRI on my swollen knee.

The results were revealing, conclusive and devastating. The tissue showed some type of cancer around the knee area.

Even though I knew this was a possibility, the finality and definitiveness of it hit me quite hard. As Dr. Fatti gently explained the diagnosis and the possibilities, I had to choke back tears and the impulse to weep.

Confirmation would have to wait for a week or so until

my appointment with the oncologist and the various tests, including a bone marrow biopsy, which he would perform.

But for the moment what was once a shadow had now become a dark cloud descending upon me. In a few weeks, I would learn about the certainty of that cloud and its nature.

Waiting

$\mathcal{D}$octor Stephen Graziano serves full time on the staff of the Regional Oncology Center, a department or division of the Upstate Medical University in Syracuse, New York. He, at the time, was also involved in research at a nearby Veteran's Administration Hospital.

I had a companion for this first appointment with Dr. Graziano. Ann Tyndall, wife of Dr. Gary and herself a nurse, was there not to hold my hand, but to drive me home following the visit. She anticipated, accurately so, that after a bone marrow biopsy, I would be told not to drive several hours because of the drugs used in connection with this procedure.

While frightened would be too strong a word, I did feel quite anxious as we walked into the center. Images of what kind of cancer affected people I would see and thoughts about what my appointment would be like certainly flooded my mind. But the staff was very friendly, competent and reassuring.

I first faced all the necessary paper work, including those complex insurance details. Next, I had to complete a lengthy form seeking my personal health history. As a nurse, friend and the spouse of my personal physician, Ann was an enormous help in filling out that extensive document. We noted there that my father had died of cancer in his forties and my mother of that same disease in her sixties.

After a nurse carried out the standard examination of height, weight, blood pressure, etc., Dr. Graziano, a relatively young, bright and highly respected oncologist, entered the examination room. Following some discussion and further checking of bodily details, he outlined his plan to proceed immediately with the bone marrow biopsy, followed by rather thorough blood tests and X-rays. The results, he said, confirming or rejecting the diagnosis of my suspected disease, would be available in several days.

Despite an outward, light-hearted manner, I know that my anxiety level about the biopsy ran high. A shot of Demerol in my upper arm helped with that as a feeling of well being soon began to seep through my body. I understand better now how some people become addicted to drugs. After numbing and preparing my back near the hip, Dr. Graziano inserted the lengthy needle and aspirated what was needed from my bone marrow.

The biopsy was not as bad an experience as anticipated, although a repeated one several weeks later seemed to be more difficult.

With the blood tests as well as additional X-rays finished and an appointment card for three weeks later in my hand, we left the building and drove away. The Demerol-induced sense of well being continued for the next two hours.

Several days later I left with three priests friends for about two weeks of vacation in San Juan, Puerto Rico. The flu type symptoms that I had been experiencing for the last week had almost run its course, but the symptoms of my cancer continued — night sweats, chills, fatigue and persistent cough. Moreover, while we knew almost certainly that I had this particular form of cancer, there would be no confirmation of it until Dr. Graziano had seen the test results and communicated with Dr. Tyndall.

For the dozen years we have been vacationing in Puerto Rico, my own pattern has changed little: late big breakfast; prayer and serious reading; an afternoon with novels (Clancy, Ludlum, Grisham, Sparks, Higgins, Follett), a late afternoon five mile run on a street by the ocean, Mass, happy hour and dinner in a local restaurant.

But for me this year, the pattern was to change. I had to walk, since my knee kept me from jogging; the cough made sleeping more difficult and conversation at dinner quite troublesome; the cancer symptoms continued; and I was waiting for a message from Dr. Tyndall about the test results.

The call came on the second day of vacation. Yes, it was this rare form of cancer. Furthermore, I would get the details during my appointment with Dr. Graziano in two weeks.

The news was not a shock, but more of a heavy realization that my life would now be altered forever. Since I was on vacation, there were ample moments to reflect upon what all of this meant.

I occasionally wept by myself (only one of my companions knew about the cancer situation), or felt a few tears running down my face, or momentarily choked up. There never was or has been any sense of great anger at the development or real denial of the disease. But the tears and sadness puzzled me. However, friends and parishioners know from frequent observations that I easily choke up or shed tears when experiencing instances of loss or separation (sadness) and the correlative situations of reunion or oneness (joy). Such situations in movies, novels and life easily prompt within me such a choked up, often tearful response.

A friend who is also a therapist wonders if my father's departure from my mother when I was only two and the sense of multiple losses through that event might be behind this sensitivity to such loss/reunion experiences.

Whatever the deeper explanation, the fact is I respond emotionally now and then when pondering by myself the loss dimensions of cancer or when someone extends to me loving support during these recovery days.

The dark cloud of cancer, even though a less aggressive form, now was a certainty. After having had a chance to reflect upon that in a vacation environment for two weeks, the waiting was about to be over. In a few days I would know more precisely the nature of this dark cloud and its impact upon my future.

Bad News/Good News

On the Tuesday afternoon after my return from vacation, I sat down for appointment number two with the oncologist, Dr. Stephen Graziano.

He was certainly prepared and ready.

He had reviewed the blood tests, the bone marrow biopsy results and the extensive X-rays.

He had examined the X-ray and MRI film of my knee sent to him by the orthopedic specialist.

He had studied all the documentation of Dr. Tyndall's efforts on my behalf prior to connecting with the oncologist.

He had ordered a CAT scan for my chest and abdomen to be certain there were no signs of cancer in those locations.

He intended to do a second bone marrow biopsy on me that afternoon for additional needed data.

He had consulted with the other oncologists on staff about my case.

He had made copies of a lengthy medical journal report discussing my disease.

Now he was ready to give me the diagnosis.

I am certain that all or most oncologists follow a similar procedure of extensive tests before reaching their conclusions.

However, I found it gave and gives me confidence to have as my cancer physician an experienced oncologist also doing research at a medical center. That background would indicate he is on top of current developments and aware of the latest findings. Having all the testing processes available either at the Regional Oncology Center (ROC) or next door at the connected hospital also made matters much more convenient in many ways.

His words were gracious, but to the point:

"Father, it would appear you have Waldenstrom's Macroglobulinemia, a rare form of bone marrow cancer. It is the least aggressive and most indolent of those types of cancer. It is also both treatable and rather easily treatable. While it is incurable, the success rate of treatment is quite high and the average years of survival run between 5-7 years, although that average could be much longer or even shorter. Only about 1500 cases are diagnosed each year in the United States, mostly affecting patients over 65. It has been seven years since I have treated a case of Waldenstrom's disease."

While his clear diagnosis was not unexpected, its definitiveness seemed to stun me a bit and became a kind of reality check.

In retrospect, I saw this as a classic bad news/good news statement.

The *bad news* was that I surely had cancer; that it would never go away; that for the rest of my life I will be visiting a doctor and having tests on a regular basis; that while treatment probably will reduce and contain the evil invader, it will always be there ready to break out in a destructive way; that it is treatable, but nevertheless incurable; that in a certain fashion I will in this life be always a sick man with certain limitations.

These thoughts about the future were hard to take for one who has been extremely healthy throughout his life, has not ever experienced a headache and never taken an adult aspirin. Adjusting to that bad news would require time and patience.

The *good news* was that Waldenstrom's disease (I never could spell or pronounce that second word) is treatable; that the treatment is relatively easy compared to other types of cancer; that the prospects of the therapy curing the current symptoms (fatigue and cough) and containing the cancer are excellent; that the treatment while slow working should within a year restore much of my former energy and free breathing; that future tests and physician visits will probably be less frequent than present; that I should be able to work, even though at a lower level, while undergoing therapy.

After I had an opportunity to absorb his diagnosis and pose a few questions, Dr. Graziano then outlined the treatment.

About once a month I would daily take 11 tablets (Leukeran 2mg) for a week, followed by several weeks of non-pill taking and recuperation. I would have a blood test every other week at the ROC and return to see him in 4-6 weeks. After reviewing the next test results, he will then prescribe another dosage and the process will be repeated. That therapy procedure should continue for about a year.

After he had completed the second bone marrow biopsy, I left ROC with two prescriptions in my pocket — one for the 77 (11 x 7) potent pills and the other for medicine in case there was nausea or vomiting while taking the chemotherapy.

That night Dr. Tyndall, his wife Ann and I had dinner at

a local restaurant to process this experience and plan how to convey the results to others.

During the previous months of sickness, testing and speculation, only a few trusted friends knew of my condition. Many, of course, had heard the ugly cough and observed my deteriorating energy, but had no idea something more serious might be behind them. Looking backwards, I realize this kind of secrecy was a very wise move and eliminated all kinds of false rumors and useless worries.

Now, however, it was time to make public what had been private.

We decided first to inform at a morning meeting all the Cathedral team or staff and, that same night, to share that information with the Parish Pastoral Council. The following weekend, at all the Masses, we would disclose details of my sickness to parishioners and visitors who happened to be with us over those two days. I also decided that night at dinner to absent myself from pastoral work (Masses, sacramental rites, appointments, calls) at the Cathedral for around a month or so (actually most of Lent until Holy Week).

We made the weekend announcement in a unique, but I think very effective way. The next chapter will describe how we did this.

Public Disclosure

We had to postpone the pill-taking and public announcement of my cancer for ten days.

My priest partner in the parish was away on a well-deserved week of vacation. In his absence, I needed to cover the Cathedral, including two funerals which occurred during that period. We also were hosting the first annual "Sweet Cabaret," a fund raiser for our school kids due to attract over 400 participants. I wanted to be there and, as much as possible, be at the top of my game.

The weekend of Masses for this public disclosure was simultaneously to be my first weekend away from the parish. A long time friend, Father Michael Donovan, had agreed to take me in as a part-time guest when I was not at the Cathedral. Consequently, on that Saturday afternoon before the announcement, I packed my bags and drove the twenty minutes to Marcellus and St. Francis Xavier Church, my sometimes home away from home for the next month.

Dr. Gary Tyndall spoke during homily time at all the Cathedral's weekend Masses, explaining in detail my health situation. I could not have had a more perfect person for this task. A tall and strapping man, an active parishioner and eucharistic minister, director of the Veteran's Administration Hospital Emergency Room, my personal friend and physician for about a dozen years, Gary automatically commanded the people's attention and addressed them with knowledgeable authority.

First, however, he read this introductory statement from me to the people at Mass.

The Church through the Scriptures gives us some pertinent messages for our spiritual life on this Second Sunday of Lent here at the Cathedral as we prepare for Easter.

From the Hebrew Scriptures or the Old Testament, the Church points out Abraham as our Father in Faith. The second stained glass window on the Jefferson Street side features Abraham. God told him to leave his comfortable home for an unknown land. He did so with faith and trust that God would take care of him in the future.

Paul, speaking to his protégé and colleague Timothy, tells him that he must bear a share of the hardship which the Gospel entails.

The Gospel is a Gospel of hope. In the transfiguration, Christ, transformed with garments white as snow and face shining as the sun, offered his close friends a prediction that while he would suffer, he would emerge victorious.

He offers the same promise to us.

These readings have a particular significance for me and for all of us at the Cathedral this weekend. Dr. Gary

Tyndall, his wife Ann and their two young adult children, Julie at Binghamton University and Megan, a high school sophomore very active here at the Cathedral, have been friends of mine for a dozen years, involved parishioners at the Cathedral for a half dozen years and Dr. Gary has been my personal physician over those dozen years. I have asked him to give a report on my current health situation. Naturally, I am most grateful to him for doing this.

Then Dr. Tyndall presented his own lengthy description of my health condition:

Over the past three or four months it's been obvious that Father Champlin has had some health problems that have been difficult for him and those around him to bear.

My presentation will consist of three parts; the presentation and investigation of his complaints, his diagnosis and an outline of his current treatment plan and the expectations regarding that plan.

I. Presentation

In September of 2000 Father Champlin began to have some problems with numbness along the left side of his chin. He had a history of significant arthritis in his cervical spine, had been doing a lot of writing and we felt that the persistent writing was aggravating the condition. I asked one of the neurologists in town to take a look at him to be sure we weren't missing something more significant.

He was seen in the office, underwent a thorough exam, had blood work and several radiological tests done to investigate the complaint further. An MRI of his cervical spine done at the time showed the persistent arthritis in the cervical spine, but it also showed an abnormality in a couple of his thoracic vertebral bodies. He also had a MRI of his brain and this showed a couple of areas in his skull that were of concern. The radiologists suggested that the picture was consistent with metastatic cancer, particularly prostatic cancer. Since his exam and blood test for prostate cancer had been normal for years, this was not thought to be a possibility. He underwent a bone scan at that time to further investigate the abnormalities found on the MRI, and it was normal. All of his blood work was also normal. We then ordered a serum protein electrophoresis, a special blood test that can measure the amounts of each type of antibody that we normally produce.

Antibodies are substances our bodies make to fight infection. Sometimes one of the cells that make these antibodies can become a cancer and produce this antibody in excess. This test showed a small spike in one of the light chains for the IgM antibody of this profile. This could be caused by a condition known as MGUS (monoclonal gammopathy of uncertain significance), or by an entity related to myeloma called Waldenstrom's Macroglobulinemia.

During this time his initial complaint of numbness along his chin disappeared and never returned.

The next step in his evaluation involved seeing a specialist in hematology/oncology to have a bone marrow test completed. These arrangements were made. However, after much thought and prayer, Fr. Champlin decided to cancel the appointment and made an informed decision to watch and wait.

He did well until May of 2001 when he became fatigued and short of breath while running in the annual Memorial Day race in Camillus. He actually had to stop twice, something he had never done in his 30+ years of running. He was seen by a cardiologist in Syracuse, underwent a stress test, which he completed without difficulty, and the episode was shrugged off as dehydration. He continued to run without difficulty.

In October of 2001 he developed an upper respiratory illness that had as one of its features a nagging and persistent dry cough. Blood work and X-rays were normal and he was treated with antibiotics without improvement. The cough was particularly disturbing to him because it affected his ability to speak in public. He was also beginning to feel tired and drained early in the day, requiring longer naps to recover.

It was decided to repeat his blood work. The repeat studies showed that his spike had risen 5 fold to 1600mgs/dl. We were successful in convincing him to see a specialist and at least hear what they had to say about further workup, which would involve a bone marrow examination.

Around this time he began to have problems with pain in one of his knees after running.

He saw Dr. Fatti an orthopedic surgeon and long time friend; X-rays were negative and he was placed on an anti-inflammatory medication and an icing regimen after running. A complication soon developed. I spoke with Dr. Fatti, advised him of the possible problems with his blood, who then ordered an MRI. This was clearly abnormal, showing some infiltration of areas of his bone marrow. Dr. Fatti was instrumental in encouraging him to see the oncologist with whom an appointment had already been made.

He has seen Dr. Steven Graziano of the Regional Oncology Center at SUNY Health Science Center in Syracuse. They seemed to connect instantly. He underwent the bone marrow examination and it confirmed the diagnosis of Waldenstrom's Macroglobulinemia.

II. Diagnosis

Waldernstrom's Macroglobulinemia is a disorder caused by a cancer in the lymphocytes that produce IgM. Remember our earlier reference to IgM as one of the antibodies we all make to fight infection. It is a fairly uncommon cancer, with approximately 1500 cases diagnosed yearly in the U.S. usually affecting patients over the age of 65. The cause is unknown. The symptoms associated with WM are related to the amount of the circulating IgM, and to the disposition of IgM in various tissues. WM always involves the bone marrow. Depending on the degree of infiltration, patients may experience mild to severe anemia. Approximately one-third of patients possess enlarged lymph nodes, spleen and liver. Occasionally, patients with WM have been reported with lung, renal and GI involvement.

IgM is a large molecule, and two-thirds of it stays in the vascular space. As increased concentrations of this protein occur, the blood gets thicker and blood flow can become sluggish. It is characterized by fatigue, bleeding and ocular, neurologic and cardiovascular complications.

The diagnosis is made by bone marrow biopsy.

Many of you who are familiar with cancers may ask what the stage is?

WM is not classified in stages. Since it is a lymphoma and is always in the bone marrow, it would always be classified as a stage 4 disease. Also, many times the treatment would depend on the stage. In WM treatment depends on the presence or absence of symptoms. If the diagnosis is made, but the patient is not symptomatic, treatment is not given because there is no evidence to show that it prolongs survival. Treatment should only be started when there is evidence for disease progression.

III. Treatment

When patients begin to have symptoms such as anemia, weight loss, fever, night sweats or signs of the blood becoming thick, they should be treated.

Chemotherapy with chlorambucil has been the standard primary therapy for symptomatic patients. Treatment can be given as a few tablets daily, or a large number, and in Fr. Champlin's situation, 11 tablets daily for 1 week. This course is repeated every 6 weeks. Fr. Champlin completed his first week of therapy this past Friday. The response tends to be slow and often several months of therapy is required to determine the effectiveness of the medication. For patients who do not respond to initial chemotherapy, there are other drug options that have been effective in up to 80% of non–responders.

The median duration of survival is 5.4 years, with 20% of the patients living as long as 10 years. Up to one fifth of these patients die from other unrelated causes.

A few people have asked about bone marrow transplant as a treatment option. This has been accomplished in a few younger patients with disease that was not responsive to chemotherapy. However, there is not enough data to render this more than investigational at this stage.

Summary

We have reviewed the presentation, the diagnosis and recommended treatment plans for Fr. Champlin's illness.

Just a few final points need to be made.

Chemotherapy in its attempt to destroy the bad cancer cells also destroys good infection fighting cells. This is one of the reasons Fr. Champlin has decided to take a leave of absence from Cathedral activities. It is critical for the two weeks following his week of treatment that he limits his exposure to large numbers of people and potential infectious diseases. The very nature of his profession makes that impossible. His schedule will be adjusted accordingly once we determine how he is responding to his ongoing therapy.

The last point relates to his persistent cough. He is currently seeing an extremely competent pulmonary specialist at SUNY, Health Science Center, Dr. Robert Lenox. He is to undergo further testing this week. It is possible that the cough is from infiltration of his lung by the cancer, but other possibilities are also being explored.

As one would expect, the parishioners were extremely attentive, with some surprised, stunned and saddened.

Dr. Tyndall concluded by reading my final remarks:

I have some concluding remarks from Father Champlin.

Once again I want to express my gratitude to Dr. Gary

for this presentation at all the weekend Masses and also for his superb attention as my physician during these past dozen years. Father Amedeo Guida will be taking full responsibility for pastoral matters at the Cathedral such as Masses, Baptisms, funerals and similar needs. I appreciate very much his willingness to assume those tasks in my absence. Our very dedicated and efficient Cathedral team, who will keep in touch with me over this period of time, will care for the administration affairs of Cathedral.

Finally, I am anticipating with gratitude your love and support during the time ahead as well as your prayers. My greatest needs, right now, are: courage, patience and strength. Of course, we likewise pray that God, using competent health care personnel and proven medical treatments, will correct my poor health condition. My hope is to be back around Easter having taken a significant step toward containing the cancer and curing the cough.

May God bless you all.

We had decided in the planning that Gary would exit immediately after his presentation, lest he be bombarded with questions.

There were several reasons for this method for announcing my cancer condition.

First, if I had been the one to disclose this information, it would have been no doubt for me and perhaps for others a tearful experience.

Second, it provided parishioners with an informed, accurate, and authoritative explanation of my condition.

Third, it eliminated rumors and guesswork. Even so, people told me that they had heard stories about my having terminal cancer or dying at a local hospital.

Fourth, it treated the parish as a family, keeping it aware and knowledgeable about the health of one of its members and enlisting their loving, prayerful support.

We did, I think, the right thing and in the right way.

Gary has a new respect for all Catholic clergy. He realizes now just how taxing is the task of preaching at multiple Masses over a weekend and how welcome is an afternoon nap prior to the early Sunday evening Mass.

While this public disclosure was happening at the Cathedral, I was eating, or actually half-starved, devouring my first regular meal in a week at the Marcellus parish. I had just completed seven difficult days of the first treatment, those 77 chemo pills or eleven daily for a week, had lost 15 pounds and was very hungry.

A Sick Puppy

I left the oncologist after my second appointment with a prescription for two pills and a clear diagnosis of the disease and its treatment. He had given me long-term hope, but naturally no immediate relief. Consequently, I still was suffering the multiple symptoms of that cancer. A description of them follows, although neither in chronological sequence nor in rank of their discomfort.

Night sweats. I initially became aware of this phenomenon on vacation in Puerto Rico. Every morning my pajamas were damp with moisture, although not soaked in sweat, and after several days they reeked. Dr. Tyndall informed me that this was both a symptom and common effect of the cancer.

Chills. The chills seemed to begin upon my return home. They would surface on occasion when I felt fatigue creeping in or just didn't feel well. The remedy paralleled my past experiences with flu. The only comfortable or desirable place during those bouts with influenza seemingly was in bed. So, here, with the onset of the chills, I would retreat to my bedroom, climb on top of the covers, and pull up a blanket or quilt over me. The chills and the shaking would stop in a few minutes and then I would slip into a deep sleep for an hour or so. Fortunately, their frequency and intensity diminished soon after my treatment started.

Fatigue. As earlier noted, during the past year I experienced a growth in fatigue and a decrease in energy. However, that now became much more pronounced. I felt shaky during a Mass and exhausted afterwards. It was a struggle to simply get through the two funeral liturgies of that first week after the diagnosis. I could do some office work, but the doing required real effort. After a few hours my body quite emphatically would tell me once and usually twice daily that it would function no longer unless I immediately took a nap. Without any protest and quite willingly I would retreat upstairs and swiftly fall into a hard sleep for one or two hours. A five-mile walk left me totally depleted.

Cough. In October, I contracted an ugly and deep, but dry cough. There was no congestion or expectoration, but these frequent coughs drained what little energy I had. The companion shortness of breath likewise made preaching or speaking and celebration of Mass a burdensome challenge. Visits with people in the parish office were also punctuated with frequent coughs which surely were troublesome to them. I could no longer sing the priest's parts of the Mass. This shortness of breath made climbing stairs difficult and jogging nearly impossible. At that time, too, the coughing would delay my "instant" sleep pattern and sometime interrupt the sleep itself. In a word, the cough was debilitating to me and I presume disturbing to others. It was particularly the persistent cough that led me to absent myself from contact with people for the first month of treatment.

Because of the cough's persistence, my physician arranged for me to see Dr. Robert Lenox, a pulmonary specialist also on the staff of the Health Science Center and the Upstate Medical University. I found his reputation as an extremely competent physician to be well justified. He was also gracious, thorough and definite.

At our first meeting he commented, "I don't believe cancer is behind your dry cough. Those kind of persistent coughs are usually caused by allergies, reflux (acid from foods returning to agitate the bronchial system) or asthma."

However, Dr. Lenox, knowing I was already scheduled for a CAT scan of my chest and abdomen, ordered a breathing test for me at the hospital. He then scheduled an appointment after the results of those procedures were available.

I underwent the CAT scan immediately after completing my first week-long dosage of chemo pills. Preliminary instructions indicated that I was to have nothing to eat or drink three hours beforehand. Upon arrival at the hospital, the receptionist told me I needed to consume two bottles of liquid essential for the procedure.

"Nurse, I just finished a week of chemo pills and my stomach is still rather unsettled."

"Well, do the best you can. Which taste do you prefer pineapple, apple or orange?"

I selected the pineapple flavor and gingerly sipped the contents.

A half hour later I was ushered into the procedure area, discarded most of my clothes and put on the flimsy, loose-fitting robe for the scan.

As I was lying on the apparatus waiting to be pushed into the cylinder, a nurse or resident doctor came to my side and in broken English told me she was going to inject dye into my vein for the scan. Ouch! I hadn't expected this dimension of the procedure.

She then explained that I might feel warm or flushed and would want to pee, but couldn't. "What was that?" I asked.

"You will want to pee, but can't."

I inwardly chuckled at her word choice and this interesting bit of conflictual guidance.

After the 20 or so minutes on the table, I was pulled out and disengaged. At that time, a technician came around from his protective barrier and asked: "Aren't you on the radio? You may have tried everything else. Why not try God?"

For over a year I have been doing a 60-second radio spot called, "Spiritual Suggestions for a Stress-Filled Society." The messages occur at 5:43 P.M. (paid, prime drive time) Monday, Wednesday and Friday on a local news and talk station. They are repeated as public service announcements perhaps 70 times that week at different hours during the day or night. The message is definitely spiritual but so crafted that Christians, Jews, and Muslims and other believers find them acceptable.

I do not have hard figures about my listening audience, but the frequency of comments, "I heard your radio spot" or "I like your radio message" is most encouraging.

Each spot concludes, "You may have tried everything else, why not try God."

The CAT scan technician obviously is one of my listeners.

The breathing test, also conveniently at the hospital, took place in a remarkably small room of that large building.

The patient sits in a kind of cage and several times breathes into a circular tube. The computer records the results. My persistent cough made this exercise almost impossible, and as expected, the printout revealed my currently below par lung capacity.

The obviously keen, experienced and dedicated tester finally had me inhale a medicated mist. He almost jumped out of his seat as he pointed to his assistant the computer's recording of my reaction. The sudden improvement in my lung capacity and breathing ability seemed significant.

He later talked on the phone with Dr. Lenox and obviously sent the results to him.

Several days later I had my second appointment with pulmonary specialist Dr. Lenox.

He summarized results of the text and outlined a plan of action.

"I have been doing more research and discovered that there have been incidences of cancer in the bronchial area with patients who have Waldenstrom's disease. So that might be the case here."

"The CAT scan showed both chest and abdomen are clear. Your breathing test indicated that your lung capacity at present is far below normal, but that you responded well to the medication mist."

"I am giving you a prescription for two medicated inhalers which you are to use twice a day for a month. If you do not feel better in a week, please call me. My assistant will instruct you as how to use those inhalers."

I walked back to my residence feeling a bit of encouragement for the first time. I should feel better in a week's time, he had predicted, and I did.

Before my second visit to Dr. Lenox and his prediction of improvement, I had to suffer the dark and difficult week of dosage #1 with the 77 pills.

Dr. Graziano had said that I might get sick to my stomach and urged use of the prescribed pills in those circumstances. I also assumed and learned that those anti-nausea and vomiting pills had a negative side effect. His warning and recommendation made me a bit weary of this chemo pill taking procedure.

Dr. Tyndall suggested I take four in the early morning, three later in the morning and four at noon — all with a little food. I obediently followed his recommendations.

Even though I still suffered the chills, night sweats, fatigue and cough, there were no noticeable impacts of the chemo over the first two days. I ate very lightly and certainly felt anxious about the possible nausea.

Then the toxic pills (which kill both the bad cells and good cells as well as upsetting one's bodily system) began their work.

I felt more fatigued. I felt somewhat nauseated. I felt uneasy and sick and anxious.

About day four, Dr. Tyndall remarked that I probably was through the crisis time and would not get sick. Wrong!

That evening our cook at my request prepared tomato soup for me. I probably consumed it and the crackers too rapidly. I left the table in good condition, but within minutes knew what was coming and made a dash for the bathroom, arriving there almost in time.

The wrenching experience brought back memories of childhood when I knelt by the toilet bowl with mom holding a cold wash towel on my forehead.

I was indeed a sick puppy that night. The oncologist indicated I should be drinking 6-8 full glasses of fluids each day while taking the pills. Here I was not even able to hold anything down and would now be dehydrated. I was also fatigued and hungry and down in the dumps about the whole process. A friend who called that night could tell by my voice just how discouraged I was.

The next day, the Tyndalls suggested that I take the anti-nausea pills before breakfast and later in the morning. I can't remember the effect of the pills but was able to eat small amounts for the rest of the dosage period without another vomiting episode. I continued to feel weary (an effect of the chemo as well as the disease), somewhat nauseated and just not comfortable.

However, Friday came — the last day of the pills and I survived, although 15 pounds lighter and probably depressed by the experience. Nevertheless, normalcy returned rather quickly. I ate heartily that first main meal on Saturday night and on Sunday evening at a restaurant hungrily consumed rolls, salad, a steak dinner and hot fudge sundae.

I gradually regained some of the weight. Moreover, my stomach and internal systems soon were functioning in normal fashion.

Most significantly, however, both my fatigue and cough lessened a bit. There was hope now and a light at the end of the tunnel. But prior to this, during those sick puppy days and even before, I did some serious reflecting and praying about this sickness, disease or cancer and its meaning for my life.

Absorbed

_M_onths before he died, the late Joseph Cardinal Bernardin of Chicago wrote his personal reflections in a small book entitled _The Gift of Peace_. In it he described his initial bout with cancer and the second encounter with that disease which led to his death.

Between those two accounts, the bishop described a more painful experience, the false accusation that he had sexually molested a young man named Steven Cook while Cook was a seminarian in Cincinnati. The charge startled and devastated Cardinal Bernardin and the widespread media coverage marred his reputation.

Eventually Cook, now afflicted with AIDS, recanted and asked that the charges be withdrawn. Subsequently, the Cardinal initiated and carried out a very moving reconciliation with the afflicted man. They continued occasional contact by phone and mail until Steven's death shortly thereafter.

Cardinal Bernardin took great pride in his penmanship. In a very clever bit of editing, the book's personal introductory letter as well as the chapter titles, reflecting that writing skill, are done in his own clear and attractive hand script. _The Gift of Love_, published after the cardinal's death, became a national best seller, first in hard cover and now in paperback.

His basic theme and suggestion for persons afflicted in any way, especially with cancer, is "letting go." If we "let go," the cardinal maintains, "if we place ourselves totally in the hands of the Lord, the good will prevail."

Cardinal Bernardin also commented that we should pray when we are well, because when we are ill, we probably won't.

That is so true. We tend to become preoccupied with our sickly condition, struggle with our aches, and wonder what the future holds for us. Prayer often becomes impossible or takes a back seat for us.

This has not exactly been the case for me, especially in the beginning. For decades, as I have mentioned, I have tried to spend two hours at prayer early in the day. During that period of time, I usually offer Mass, pray part of the Liturgy of the Hours, read a chapter from the Old Testament and spend several minutes with a spiritual book, leaving a half hour for personal reflection and meditation.

Since the cancer diagnosis, I have, if anything, been even more faithful to that daily regimen.

But Cardinal Bernardin's observation struck home during the ten-day period when I was sick as a puppy with the cancer symptoms and the side effects of the chemotherapy.

I found myself totally absorbed with my illness, entirely oblivious of anyone or anything beyond myself. I felt so terrible, so ill that nothing else crossed my mind. I wondered how long this would last, would I ever feel healthy again. I continued the formal prayers, but my mind was focused totally upon myself and my sickness.

The words of the Catholic Church's ritual for the *Pastoral Care of the Sick* now took on a new meaning for me. It stresses that "we should fight strenuously against all sickness" (a frequent theme of the many get-well cards I received). It also teaches that "those who are seriously ill need the special help of God's grace lest they be broken in spirit and, under the pressure of temptation, become broken in spirit." The ritual then reminds us that the Sacrament for the Anointing of the Sick provides unique help for the seriously ill so they will be "able not only to bear suffering bravely, but also to fight against it."

Once the sick as a puppy period passed the absorption with my sorry state likewise disappeared or at least diminished. Now my mind cleared a bit and I pondered in prayer issues like these:

My cancer is treatable, but incurable. That means I will have this disease for the rest of my life, will have regular blood tests and appointments with an oncologist, and probably will require occasional treatment when the cancerous presence acts up.

Is this actually a preparation for my death or a sickness which will pass?

Will the fatigue eventually diminish and my former energy return?

Even if the treatment, as projected, succeeds, my future, according to the statistics, will be probably 5-7 years. That means at 72, I can anticipate the end of my time here on earth to be at around 77-79 years of age.

How much will I need to adjust my schedule of work to accommodate my future limited energies? Can I, for example, deal with those multiple Saturday weddings during the marrying season?

If I do recover well, is that God's sign that I am to spend my remaining days actively serving others? What about retirement or at least resignation as a pastor/rector of the Cathedral?

How can I best use the remaining years of my life in this world?

The Focalare Movement, founded in Italy by Chiara Lubich during World War II, provided a spiritual attitude for dealing with my most burdensome symptoms: the persistent fatigue and shortness of breath.

Those in the movement usually radiate a real joy, part of which flows from their approach toward suffering. Whatever the pain or problem, they seek immediately to refer this difficulty to the abandoned, deserted Christ on the cross. It links them with the suffering Savior.

In quiet moments, I often reflect upon that approach. Christ must have felt great weariness and fatigue from the arrest on Holy Thursday through his death on the cross. My own fatigue connects me with this dimension of the Savior's suffering. Jesus probably died by suffocation, his suspended arms on the cross no longer able to sustain his sagging body. He could breathe no more. My dry cough and shortness of breath similarly links me with the Lord on Calvary.

Throughout the day, I seldom explicitly recall those connections of continued fatigue and shortness of breath to the abandoned, deserted one on the cross. But I regularly do remember them during my reflective prayer periods.

In the early stages of my illness and especially at those very sick moments my thoughts turned now and then to life after death, to eternity, to what the next world will be like and how well or poorly prepared I am for that destiny.

Eternal Life and Temporary Conversions

*A*s Dr. Tyndall mentioned in his public disclosure, I had a temporary cancer scare a year before the Camillus race. Tests conducted for another situation indicated the possibility of a tumor or cancer in the brain and prostate.

The news was indeed a jolt. All of my various examinations, tests and X-rays of the past disclosed no problems and, in fact, would characterize me as an unusually healthy older man.

This was so unexpected.

There was some weeping and sadness by myself and with friends over the prognosis. But it also prompted some soul-searching on my part.

Should I clean up my cluttered room and office? Have I completed the funeral arrangement form requested by the diocese? Are my financial affairs in order? Am I ready to meet God? What changes should I make in my way of living now?

Thanks to the influence of Dr. Tyndall, I did not experience an excruciating wait of a week or longer for the bone scan ordered to verify or discount the presence of brain and prostate cancer. It was arranged for the following afternoon.

Dr. Tyndall learned the results of this bone scan almost

immediately and telephoned me indicating that there were no signs of the cancers. Apparently the earlier test was flawed in that regard.

We were, naturally, greatly relieved and grateful. However, I noticed something rather definite happened. The intensity of my introspection instantly vanished; life went back to normal; the resolutions were seemingly forgotten; and any contemplated conversion of lifestyle slipped from my consciousness.

Did I clean up my room and office? No. Did I complete the funeral arrangement form? Yes. Did I put my financial affairs in order? Perhaps a bit. Did I continue to concentrate more intently on meeting God or improving my lifestyle? Not really.

I was surprised by the swiftness of this shift from serious preoccupation with eternal life and its ramifications to a rapid resumption of life as usual here on earth.

Such swift shifts, I think, are probably not uncommon. Faced with some ominous crisis, we may make secret deals with God, promises to change our lives, vows to undergo a personal conversion in our lifestyles. But when the potential disaster rather quickly passes us by, those deals, promises and conversions likewise seem to pass away. They were temporary conversions, valid for a short time only. Interestingly, the Latin root of the word temporary, *tempus*, means time.

One can imagine addictive smokers warned by a physician after an examination that they may have cancerous spots on their lungs. The addicts instantly promise God and others that they will never smoke again and perhaps will also go to church, be good to the poor and love their spouses.

At a subsequent appointment the doctor informs them that these were false alarms, that succeeding tests showed no signs of cancer, that the spots had vanished. The relieved patient quickly asks: "Doctor, do you have a cigarette?"

But these crisis-prompted conversions or inner changes are not always just temporary. An older man, not a Roman Catholic, worships at Mass with us every weekday almost without fail. As a very a young soldier he landed in Korea, witnessed the kind of armed warfare in which he was about to engage, and with great anxiety said to God: "If you protect me here, save me from this mess and get me home safely, I will go to church every Sunday." And he has.

Later, struggling with prostate cancer, he again turned to God and vowed: "If I survive this, I will try to be as good, as perfect as I can be." He admits that he hasn't succeeded totally in his resolutions, but he consciously tries always to do what is right. Praying in our church each day probably is part of that response to his conversion promise.

In the early days of my illness and treatment, I found myself once more thinking rather intensely about eternal life and my current time on earth. Since the tests now revealed that the cancer was real, I received no sudden relief message. Moreover, my prospects, while not bleak, were sobering.

I can't state that there have been since then great conversions or major adjustments in my life. But, at least at this time, five months since the diagnosis, some inner changes have occurred. With improvement in my health, the intensity of reflection has diminished. However, I think I am praying more attentively, have tried to deal with some issues that impede my relationship with God and am more conscious that my time on this earth has rather circumscribed limits. This last awareness exerts a subtle, and perhaps not so subtle, effect upon the choices I make.

During those low moments early on — the combination of the chemo treatment and the cancer symptoms — I did find myself in prayer reflecting quite specifically upon eternity, upon life after death, upon what I might expect in the next world.

I suppose it was only natural that those thoughts or reflections would reflect the content of my many funeral homilies over the years. These always include a brief sketch of our hoped-for destiny, what may be the nature of heaven or eternity for us. Those concepts, sketched below, derive from our Roman Catholic biblical, liturgical and devotional traditions.

We will see God face to face.

Certain prayers at Mass, echoing the scriptural words of John, are specific about this. "There we hope to share in your glory when every tear will be wiped away. On that day we shall see you, our God, as you are. We shall become like you and praise you forever through Christ our Lord, from whom all good things come." (Eucharistic Prayer III).

For most of us, this element of heaven may not seem that humanly satisfying or attractive. But St. Augustine's famous dictum, "Our hearts are restless, O God, and will not rest until they rest in you," places this dimension of eternity in a different perspective. So, too, the human longing for perfect happiness and the frequent frustrations of everyday life may likewise expand our appreciation of seeing God face to face.

Ever since Raymond Moody in his 1976 pivotal *Life After Life* book described the similar Near Death Experiences (NDE) of several people, these phenomena have become much more widely publicized. Ron Wooten Green, a hospice chaplain, recounts a series of these in his 2001 publication, *When the*

Dying Speak. Those stories create a warm and inviting picture of personal encounters with the eternal God.

For example, Darin, a forty-nine-year-old Vietnam veteran dying of massive cancers probably caused by Agent Orange, explained to his wife Karen that he had seen next to him his deceased grandmother, four buddies killed in Vietnam, and Jesus. "They are waiting for me."

Karen did not seemed alarmed or surprised by what her husband was saying. She told the chaplain: "I've been there. You see I had an NDE years ago when I was fifteen. I went through this tunnel. A warm light kept getting stronger and stronger, brighter and brighter, more and more comforting. I saw this beautiful garden. I just wanted to stay right there."

The chaplain inquired why she came back.

"Because Jesus told me I had work to do. I pleaded with him to let me stay, but he kept telling me to go back; and he gradually disappeared. I woke up finally in a hospital room."

Darin's mother then admitted for the first time to another person that she had a similar NDE when she was thirty-four. Remembrance of that vision comforted her as she watched her dying son.

> You know, I don't want my son to die, but I think I can let him go now. I will miss him, but I have a pretty good idea of what lies ahead of him…. Darin is ready to go. His buddies, my mom, Jesus, are all waiting for him. (Chapter 8, pages 141-143).

There will be a reunion with all those we have loved and with others.

In another Mass text, a prayer reads: "Make us worthy to

share eternal life with Mary, the virgin mother of God, with the apostles, and with all the saints who have done your will throughout the ages. May we praise you in union with them, and give you glory through your Son, Jesus Christ." (Eucharistic Prayer II).

I am not a regular visitor of gravesites or a person who carefully remembers the death anniversaries of people close to me. Lest that sound crass and unbelieving, everyday at Mass, in the section which recalls those who have died, I explicitly name my mother, father, stepfather, grandparents, three great aunts who prayed me into the priesthood, a few others, and some recently deceased individuals.

During my short period of intense reflection on eternity, I recall, probably for the first time, reflecting quite vividly upon being in heaven with my mother and stepfather, my father (whom I never knew since he left home when I was about two) and those other persons I mentioned.

As my condition improved and I resumed work, those ruminations also faded into the background.

Our sorrows and pains will cease.

Families frequently select a passage from the Book of Revelation for the funeral service which speaks specifically about the end of all tears and suffering:

> This is God's dwelling among men. He shall dwell with them and they shall be his people and he shall be their God who is always with them. He shall wipe away every tear from their eyes, and there shall be no more death or mourning, crying out or pain, for the former world has passed away. (Revelation 21:3-4)

In comparison with other cancer victims, my present struggle with Waldenstrom's disease is like child's play, a piece of cake. As noted earlier, treatment involves simply consuming at home about once a month a quantity of chemo pills. While they do produce some discomforting side effects, these are relatively minor compared to what many others endure.

There has been no surgery, no hospitalization, no tubular infusion of potent chemicals, no intense pain.

During my priestly ministry since 1956, I have been at the bedside of countless men and women suffering enormous physical and emotional distress as they near death. For them and for their caretakers, the vision of eternal life with its immediate cessation of agonies and the eventual transformation of our bodies has been most comforting.

We will be connected in a real, but mysterious way
through love with those still on earth.

The Communion of Saints means that there is an intimate, spiritual bond between those of us here on earth living in time and those of the world to come living in eternity. They continue to love us and help us by their prayers; we can also connect with them through our love and prayers.

On the feast of All Saints, the Opening Prayer speaks of this connection: "Today we rejoice in the men and women of every time and place. May their prayers bring us your forgiveness and love." The preface for that feast contains similar thoughts: "Around your throne the saints, our brothers and sisters, sing your praise forever. Their glory fills us with joy, and their communion with us in your Church gives us inspiration and strength, as we hasten on our pilgrimage of faith, eager to meet them."

In her novel *Charming Billy*, award-winning author Alice McDermott translates the Communion of Saints to the life of Dennis whose wife was dying of lung cancer:

> It made it easier that they both believed in the simplest kind of afterlife — that my father could say to her, even in those last days, joking but without irony, "You're going to get tired of hearing from me. I'll be asking you for this, that and the other thing twenty-four hours a day. *Jesus*, you'll be saying, here comes another prayer from Dennis." And my mother would reply, her voice hoarse with pain, "Jesus might advise you to take in a movie once in a while. Give your poor wife a rest. She's in heaven, after all." (Page 45)

How much would these personal reflections on eternity impact my life? Will the conversions, the changes proposed for my lifestyle be temporary only or relatively permanent? The proof, of course, would be in the pudding. With the cough slightly diminished and the fatigue lessened somewhat, I now had an opportunity to put these new ideas into practice as I returned on a limited basis to work and the healing process continued.

The Healing Process
Continues

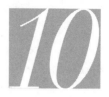

*T*he initial part of my healing process centered around tests and diagnoses by two specialists, a week of chemotherapy through pills, and inhalers used twice daily.

Shortly thereafter, I appeared to improve a bit — my fatigue had slightly declined and the cough had somewhat diminished.

Now began the longer-term healing process which included these elements:

1. *Isolation.* On that evening dinner with the Tyndalls when we planned the public disclosure of my cancer, I decided that it was necessary for me to break off contact with Cathedral parishioners. My cough, I reasoned, would not immediately disappear or even get slightly better. In about a month, I had hopes that some significant improvement would happen. Until then, I thought that people should be spared the incessant coughing.

Two steps made this people isolation possible: my hideaway room in Marcellus and a protective approach by the Cathedral team.

Father Michael Donovan, pastor of St. Francis Church in Marcellus and I have been close friends and vacationing part-

ners for three decades. He conceals a very spiritual, unselfish
and sensitive heart by his earthy sense of humor.

When I called about staying at his rectory on occasion over
several weeks, he, typical of that unselfishness, swiftly agreed.
During the next few days he and his staff arranged a perfect
second floor hideaway for me with bed, desk, reclining chair,
television and private bath.

I took advantage of that hospitality mostly on weekends
so I would not be interacting with parishioners at the Cathedral. Father Donovan also shielded me from his people in
Marcellus, many of whom I knew from the past. At the end of
the Saturday or Sunday Mass at which I was concelebrating,
he mentioned that my cancer treatment left me vulnerable to
other diseases. For that reason, he said it would be best if people
did not approach me. Moreover, I usually left the church immediately following Mass.

His receptionist also told callers that I simply was either
not there or unavailable.

It was an ideal arrangement. While at Marcellus I rested,
read and prayed. I also went out into the country for five mile
walks on several occasions (the first time totally exhausted at
the end; after the others, simply tired).

The other part of the isolation picture took place at the
Cathedral.

My partner, Father Amedeo Guida, willingly shouldered
the burden of pastoral matters — funerals, weddings, care of
the sick and personal visitations at the Parish Office.

Other priests, retired or in office functions at the Chan-
cery, assisted with Masses.

But I basically continued responsibility for administrative
matters.

The competent Cathedral team helped make this feasible. They assumed many tasks I had performed and shielded me from phone calls or people at the door.

Consequently, I was able to take care of desk work and other details, but without the energy depleting exchange with people. For the most part I still lived at the Cathedral, although few people knew that.

Looking back, I realize this isolation was a wise step in the healing process.

It gave the medicine an opportunity to work; it reduced the danger of exposure to other infections or diseases; above all, it provided me with the easy possibility of getting needed rest.

2. *Rest.* My personal physician throughout this period frequently warned me about the need "to get lots of rest." My body strongly reinforced his words.

After the initial dosage and the slight improvement, I felt able to return to the administrative work although on a limited scale. I didn't have to push too hard; nevertheless, it was still a struggle. I felt a heaviness in my step and a sluggishness in my actions, yet could function fairly well for a few hours.

Then my body would in exhaustion shout, "Enough." There was no negotiating here. I couldn't continue on to complete a few items. The body just refused to cooperate any further.

I then obediently and very willingly would go upstairs, climb on top of my bed and quickly drop off into a hard, deep sleep for one or two hours. Eventually, I would resurrect from the dead and resume work for a while longer. On some more difficult days, I might have two or even three of those naps.

When I returned to public ministry during Holy Week, the fatigue had lessened even more and the body's orders for rest were less emphatic. Even so, preaching at four Easter Masses, and celebrating two of them taxed my resources.

Soon after Easter, a subtle, but real shift happened. The cough continued to lessen, although it did not disappear, but for the first time in perhaps six months my energy resurfaced. I had been working, but the heaviness of foot and sluggishness of actions permeated my efforts. Now both heaviness and sluggishness suddenly disappeared.

I wasn't exactly bouncing up and down with excess energy, yet I could tell the difference. Extra sleep and naps I still needed. But the naps were shorter and not so deep. I was also able to persevere quite well through several busy days filled with multiple tasks.

The blood tests for anemia (hematocrit from 26.5 to 27.8) and for the Waldenstrom's disease (Igm from 2200 to 2090) reflected a shift with those slight numerical improvements. Apparently the medication was working.

3. *Medication*. I dreaded dosage #2 of the chemotherapy. I dreaded the sight of those 77 purple and puny, yet potent pills (11 each day, four with a little cereal at breakfast, three with more cereal and crackers at mid-morning and the final four with food at lunchtime). I dreaded the loss of appetite and weight; I dreaded the nausea even without the vomiting. I dreaded the increased fatigue; I dreaded feeling so sick.

I can't say that I dreaded the potential disappearance of my hair, since there is not much on top anyway (my father was bald when he reached his thirties). However, to protect against this possibility, I had my barber give me a very close and short haircut so that the absence would be less noticeable. To this point, not a hair on my head has vanished.

I probably had a slight dread that my still black, beautiful and bushy eyebrows would undergo a change. As yet, that has not occurred.

In reality, dosage #2 proved less dreadful than dosage #1. I knew better what to expect and had acquired a few coping skills. Regardless, I still lost about ten pounds and generally felt miserable, although able to function fairly well at work.

Eventually, I suppose, one taking such toxic medication realizes that feeling miserable during the therapy period means the medicine is working. A friend who has worked extensively with AIDS patients recalls one suffering man remarking: "I know that when I feel lousy, the medicine is doing its job."

During dosage #2, I ate sparingly about five or six times daily. The only food which seemed appealing was ice cream and consequently, at least three times each day, I had a dish of tasty French Vanilla ice cream, courtesy of friends.

While ingesting the pills, directions specifically insist that the patient consume 6-8 full glasses of fluid daily. Other friends delivered each week a thoughtful, but totally unsolicited gift: two cases of Poland Spring water in small plastic bottles. A large glass of water during the dosage seemed personally too much for me; these half-pint containers were more manageable. Because of them I was generally able to fulfill the 6-8 glass directions.

Although dosage #2's one-week ordeal was not as bad as dosage #1 (no vomiting for example), yet I still struggled to get through that period. The day after finishing the pills, for some reason, was a particularly bad one. However, I recovered almost immediately.

Normally chemo treatments weaken a patient's immune system, making the person vulnerable to infections or diseases carried by other individuals. Thus for ten days to two weeks, chemo patients try to avoid crowds — a difficult challenge for one who is a priest in pastoral work. For me, on the contrary, tests indicated that my blood counts stood high enough during the therapy that this precaution of avoiding people or crowds was unnecessary. The immune system remained operational.

As I commented above, within two weeks I felt a remarkable upswing in my health. The medicine appeared to be working. During physical training, the lead person in the army chants encouraging slogans. One is: "No Pain, No Gain." That seems to be the situation with this therapy. I needed to endure the two dreadful dosages if I was to experience the gain of substantially improved health.

4. *Lectures.* During the past two decades I have traveled on an average of 50,000 miles annually for lectures outside the diocese of Syracuse on pastoral subjects for mostly Catholic audiences. Quite providentially, there were very few of these engagements between January and April, the very time of my diagnosis, low moments and initial therapy.

The first one I felt able to fulfill came between dosage #1 and dosage #2. Fatigue was still a factor and the cough present, although less frequent and intense.

I was somewhat anxious about this one-hour presentation for the stewardship leaders in the diocese of St. Petersburg, Florida. Would the cough erupt frequently? Could I handle sixty minutes of straight speaking? How would my body react to the lengthy trips with change of flights from Syracuse to

Tampa and back (down on Tuesday afternoon, back on Wednesday night)?

Colleagues in this field and longtime friends suggested I tell the audience up front about my cancer. Moreover, there were several personal illustrations in the lecture related to the illness. Would I, as usual, choke up or get teary when speaking about my health condition?

The night before was not a perfect preparation for my morning experience. A group of college students were on break from the north, staying in the motel room next to mine. They invited their friends over for what seemed to be an all night noisy get together. There were scattered butts on the sidewalk outside the room the next morning. During the few quiet periods throughout the night I was inspired by the thought that they were probably saying the rosary, practicing a Taizé mantra or engaging in reflective prayer.

Despite my nervousness about the lecture, it went well. I did give a brief account about my cancer and the need, because of the cough, to speak more softly and slowly than usual for me. I choked up a few times when citing my illness experiences and needed to follow my text or outline rather closely. For some reason, fatigue was not a factor on either day, despite the long and delayed trips.

I repeated the same lecture about a month later in Escanaba, Michigan for the priests of the Marquette diocese. But by then my health had begun to experience that noticeable improvement I have described. This positive change was certainly brought about at least in part by the unbelievable wave of love, prayer and support which started to come my way and lift me up as soon as the cancer became known.

An Incredible Wave
of Support

When my cancer illness became public knowledge, one of our parish receptionists predicted an immediate avalanche of empathetic mail. She was absolutely correct. In my office there are now three cartons filled to overflowing with more than 1500 cards, letters and other items offering me love, prayers and support. They arrived daily by the dozen at the beginning and continue on a lesser scale even today. It made me wish that I had purchased some shares of Hallmark stock early on in the illness.

During the Christmas season when we receive a quantity of greetings there is a tendency to glance at the cards, check the senders and lay them aside. I didn't follow that pattern with these get-well communications. Often around 9:00 p.m., I would take several dozen to my room, sit down in an easy chair and carefully read their messages. That experience itself was both most affirming and inspirational.

I learned that an enormously wide variety of people were praying for me: from the retired Episcopal Bishop of Central New York who added me to his twice a day petition list to a Protestant breakfast prayer group in Carolina; from the Trappist monks south of Rochester to their affiliated monastery in the

Philippines; from the rector of the Catholic Cathedral in Seattle to longtime friends in Florida; from the Bishop of Albany to a couple in Texas at whose marriage I had officiated in the Cathedral less than a year ago. In addition, there were countless arranged prayers, family prayers and individual prayers on my behalf, many from a distance, but most from the local area.

Incredible and overwhelming are the only words I can find to describe this tidal wave of prayerful love and support.

Eddie, almost forty, flies commercial jets all over the world. He has not found a bride yet, much to the distress of his parents. However, since they and he are all Irish, that is not much of a surprise. Irish men often take their time getting to the altar.

I have been a close friend of his parents for over 30 years and naturally know this young man well. Eddie's handwritten note offered his concern and prayers, but also raised the question of suffering, good and evil in this world.

> It is times like these that I have a difficult time understanding God's grand scheme of things!
> Why is it that individuals of evil or malicious character remain relatively unscathed as they progress through life? Yet is seems the good and virtuous of this life are burdened with the pain and suffering!
> I suppose it is all part of the great mystery of our existence.

The reality, of course, is that no one, good or bad, can totally escape suffering during a lifetime on earth. Moreover, many "good" people do remain relatively unscathed in their lives and many "evil" persons do experience periods of great pain.

However, Eddie's question about suffering as relates to the good and bad in our world is perhaps the perennial challenging issue for every human being and especially for professional or non-professional philosophers.

While quite ill, my focus often centered upon Christ's suffering and the crucifix. Jesus on the cross does offer an answer, probably the best response to Eddie's inquiry. Here was an innocent man willing to give his life out of love for others; the sinless Son of God suffering and dying not only at the hands of others, but for others.

Sue lives in the suburbs and became a Roman Catholic over a dozen years ago. She wrote offering prayerful support, but also describing her own struggle with cancer, the spiritual help she receives from faith and the thoughts she entertains about the future.

> May your suffering from this affliction be forgotten as we see your healing happen in this GLORIOUS SEASON OF EASTER.
>
> I am recovering from lung cancer surgery and needed to have 40% of my lung removed. I had to have a very painful invasive and expansive surgery with a lung tube to drain the excess blood and water from my lung. It made me mindful that Our Lord suffered this without anesthesia or morphine but in the cruelest agony for His Great Love for Us, nailed to a Cross; I know the immensity of it now.
>
> The only truly real thing I had to hang on to when I discovered the cancer in January was the ever-present Lord. He was more real than anything else at that period through surgery and early recovery. The prayers

and Masses offered for me and the importance of those who love us is the most important gift of all — LOVE remains with me now as I recover.

I pray that my gift of time here in this world will be fruitful and I use it wisely. I am weak physically now and I am weak in my spirit at times but I attend a prayer group weekly as I can. I am more aware of those suffering alone.

Terri attends Mass daily at our Cathedral and hand delivered to me a greeting card which featured the Claude Monet floral painting, "Nympkeas and Agapanthes." Distributed by the Alzheimer's Association from Chicago, it contained no printed message on the inside. However, Terri then inscribed her own words, "Courage Father. Once again you inspire the flock."

She tucked inside the card a slip of paper cut out from some publication with comments about "What Cancer Cannot Do." The phrases of this author, a "Source Unknown," struck me, especially the call to courage.

> Cancer is so limited —
>> It cannot cripple love
>> It cannot shatter hope
>> It cannot corrode faith
>> It cannot destroy peace
>> It cannot kill friendship
>> It cannot suppress memories
>> It cannot silence courage
>> It cannot invade the soul
>> It cannot steal eternal life
>> It cannot conquer the spirit.

Tricia, a visiting nurse, offered her help in any way needed and, with her husband of nearly six years, sent their heartfelt thoughts and prayers my way. I had many connections with Tricia and her family over the years and found the poetic greeting on the face of their card an encouraging reminder. The poem is attributed merely to "Kristone."

> God has not promised
> skies always blue,
> flower-strewn pathways
> all our lives through;
> God has not promised
> Sun without rain,
> Joy without sorrow,
> Peace without pain.
> But God has promised
> Strength for the day,
> Rest for the labor,
> Light for the way,
> Grace for the trails,
> Help from above,
> Unfailing sympathy,
> Undying love.

Many, like Nancy, a Cathedral parishioner, sent cards indicating that she or they had arranged for prayers by religious committees in which I would be remembered. Her own communication included "A Prayer in Time of Suffering."

> Until my healing comes, Lord, give me Your grace so that I may accept my suffering. Give me Your strength so that I will not despair. Give me Your love so that my

suffering may bring me closer to You, the origin and source of all love.

Many persons maintain that we inherit as human beings a subtle and unconscious, but real tendency not to care deeply about ourselves. This translates into an inner judgment that we are not very lovable, if people really knew us. It, in effect, means we struggle with a shaky self-image.

Advocates of this seemingly negative theory or philosophy often rest their case on a series of questions for persons to answer with complete honesty. These include:

How well do you take compliments?

Do you often pick at yourself over what you have done, pointing out the flaw in an otherwise fairly perfect product?

Would you say you judge yourself by a double standard — requiring a spotless record to place a virtue by your name and insisting that one fall would remove the virtue from your name?

Do you, even if rather subconsciously, consider that you must earn another's love?

Must you always be the person in charge or the individual who does everything?

In a confrontation of some significance do you tend to be passive, aggressive or assertive?

Do you have a more than usual need to be recognized, affirmed and proud?

Are you struggling with any or at least a serious addiction?

Honest responses to these questions might lead an individual to concur with the theory about shaky self-image and that tendency deep down not to value ourselves or see ourselves as lovable.

Those theoretical speculations become real when some-one does something for us or displays a sincere concern about our well-being. Those actions are in reality deeds of love directed to us and they may trigger symptomatic inner reactions. We may feel uncomfortable or elated, overwhelmed or grateful.

Earlier in this book I mentioned the comment of our semi-retired, former steel worker custodian who one day passed on the suggestion, "Father, some people who love you feel you need more rest." In the face of this avalanche of get-well cards, he made another insightful comment, one related to these comments and questions about shaky self-images. "If you ever have doubts about being loved, you certainly can't have them now."

Over 100 of those communications included letters or lengthy comments about some positive connection they had with me in the past. Those notes proved to be even more touching than the mere massive outpouring of cards. I will speak about that moving experience in the next chapter.

Reviewing One's Life

*I*n the last chapter, I mentioned the question about picking at ourselves, that is, the tendency to focus on the flaws of an otherwise near-perfect effort.

This has a special relevance for older persons looking back over their lives. We seem to remember the bad choices, the sins, the failures of our lives; on the other hand, we tend to forget or diminish the good decisions, the virtues, the successes of our time on this earth.

"I wish I hadn't done that." "I regret very much that period of my life." "I wince at the thought of how I hurt some people by what I did."

Those statements are true regrets of real people. But these individuals could also, but generally do not, point out numerous good actions in their lives which far surpassed the bad deeds.

In a word, as we review our lives, there appears to be this common trend to recall with regret the shadow moments of the past and forget the bright points, to remember the poor choices and to ignore the good ones.

Those who have experienced Near Death Experiences almost universally speak of a warm personal being, God or Jesus reviewing their lives with them. The review, however, was very gentle and positive often reminding the persons of how they learned from this or that bad action.

Several Roman Catholic theologians would concur with that vision of God. They maintain that as soon as we repent, God forgets the bad we have done. Or, in a different phrasing, God does not even remember the evil which a penitent person has committed.

This incredible wave of support, described in the last chapter, has also provided me with a unique review of my own life, especially my 45 years as a priest. I tend to recall, wince over, and regret the bad choices, selfishness and major sins over those decades. I likewise, following the trend described above, generally have forgotten the countless good things accomplished during that nearly half-century of pastoral ministry.

As a priest at three relatively large parishes during this time period, one connects with many, many persons in various contexts. Also, as a fairly public figure in my current post at the Cathedral, I have had contact with countless additional people for diverse reasons. Upon learning I had cancer, a sizable number felt inclined to communicate their support. It is not surprising then, that cards of love, prayer and good wishes arrived at the parish office. Nevertheless, the huge response of over 1500 has been both mind-boggling and heartwarming.

However, I have been particularly touched by those over 100 individuals who wrote letters or notes recalling some way during the distant or recent past in which the exercise of my priesthood helped them. Reading these communications brought back memories, deeply moved me and often prompted tears.

It was like an anticipated review of my life, pointing out the good actions of my pastoral ministry, deeds I have long since forgotten. The experience led me to ask this question: Is that what it will be like standing before God at the end of my time here and at the start of my eternity? I also wonder how many individuals have been graced with such a unique opportunity to see the major portion of their lives pass, as it were, before their eyes while still on earth.

Some letters cited instances of our relationship early in my priesthood after ordination on that cold day in February, 1956.

> I'm ashamed it has taken me this long to thank you for the gift of baptism into our Church December 19, 1958. My faith has sustained me in good times as well as bad. I've heard nothing but good things about you for years. Your latest life experience just seems to make you stronger in faith. I'm so proud of you.

> I can honestly say you have been mentioned at every Mass I have attended since my baptism — I have attended daily Mass for many years.

> I continue to pray that He continue giving you strength to sustain you.

Others go back almost that far, but continue to the present:

> You have always been an inspiration to us from the time we were in pre-Cana, 42 years ago, to the present as you uplift us with your radio messages. Your gift with words have enlightened thousands and you have always conducted yourself as a man of God.

Being a cancer patient instantly makes you a member of this huge club with whom there is a common bond. Two letters reaching fairly far back into the past make both that connection and my priestly work with them.

The first came from a woman now legally blind, but who, nevertheless, with the help of a guide, penned these words:

> It was 31 years ago when you came to Fulton and I met you on the day before my surgery for a malignant tumor and I had to have a mastectomy. You gave me a little book "Fear Not, I Am With You."
>
> That book is with me at all times.

A widow added this note to her card which assured me of prayers arranged for my behalf with a religious community:

> So sorry you are so ill. You are in my daily prayers. I remember your kindness and help to me and my family 24 years ago when my husband Bill was dying of cancer. I have always kept you in my prayers.

These were understandably somewhat older people. However, I did receive letters, cards and notes from a surprising number of young persons. Joseph, for example, soon to enter high school penciled this brief note:

> I would just like to drop you a little note telling you that you are in my prayers and to tell you I hope you feel better. Over the past few years I have enjoyed getting notes and sending you money to support your yearly run in May. I would also like to thank you for all the things you taught me and my family in your great and thoughtful homilies. Hope to see you soon.

These communications were almost too numerous to count and certainly too many to cite in this book. Here are a few more excerpts citing good, but forgotten, deeds of the past.

"You sent me a card from Rome in 1977 when my father died; now I am sending you this card in response." (I was pastor-in-residence at the North American College in Rome 1976-77, with a year leave of absence from Holy Family Parish in Fulton).

"You heard my first confession in 20 years, bringing me the great peace and happiness I have had ever since."

"You went to see my spouse with Alzheimer's disease and he seemed so comforted by your words."

"You visited my husband in the VA hospital and he died a Catholic."

"You called at the house twenty years ago when as a young mother with two children age two and three I was overwhelmed with the news of my breast cancer."

This two-page, handwritten note from a high school senior did and does move me to tears. It includes photos of a First Communion child in white dress with veil and of a now grown-up young lady in high school:

My youngest brother and my Dad were present at last Sunday's Mass in the Cathedral, and heard the terrible news about your cancer. I wanted to write you to let you know that you are in my thoughts and prayers. Although you only knew me well at a very young age, the impact you had on me will last a lifetime. You have this amazing ability to make a little girl look forward to going to Mass every Sunday, and getting a big bear hug at the end, a tradition I promise I will never grow out of when it comes to you. You will always be in my heart and my mind, although it has been a while since I was able to see you on each consecutive Sunday afternoon. I am sure I am not the only one who has been touched by your kindness, but I wanted to let you know that no matter how trivial or small you may think you are in someone's life, in mine you mean the world. You are by far one of the greatest people I have ever and will ever get the chance to know. You are a shining example of faith, and a great role model.

Thank you for all that you have been for me, and let me know if there is anything I can do for you. I love you! And I'll keep praying.

P.S. No matter what this horrible disease may do to you, in my heart you will live forever!

My struggles with cancer are minimal compared to the major difficulties many others encounter with their disease. But they remain real struggles. However, the negative aspects of my condition certainly brought forth some wonderfully positive developments. The wave of letters with their loving, prayerful support and the one hundred notes producing this review of my life certainly stand at the top of the list.

To show their concern, numerous individuals daily ask, "How do you feel?" This is a well meaning, but complicated question which we will examine now.

How Do You Feel?

*A*ll sick persons, from those with the flu to those recuperating from surgery to those coping with cancer, are often asked this question, "How do you feel?"

The number of these inquiries is significant for every individual. However, for those whose occupations connect them with many people, the number of times this question is posed rises almost geometrically. When the sick person is also a public figure whose illness has been announced in the press or on television, as in my case, the number increases even further.

The question, while essentially a simple one, has hidden, even subconscious meanings underneath it. Moreover, responding to that inquiry appropriately requires careful thought.

When the doctor confirmed my cancer diagnosis, some said that this fact, made known, would change forever my relationship with others. The impression was that one thus becomes a marked person, an individual doomed or someone with a contagious disease.

I have not found that to be the case. As the last two chapters indicated, there has been this enormous outpouring of supportive and concerned cards and letters. Verbal assurances of love and prayers more than matched those printed greetings.

There can be, nevertheless, some uneasiness in speaking with a recently diagnosed cancer patient. I am not sure of the cause or causes behind this lack of comfortableness. Is it a wish not to be intrusive? Is it the fear or distress which the C word often causes within people? Is it a sober reminder of one's own mortality?

A reporter seeking information about my life and my cancer confessed that she almost dreaded speaking with me about this latter topic. It wasn't my intimidating personality or status that created the discomfort, but the sickness and the disease. I am not sure if even now that newspaper writer understands why she felt the way she did.

Some consider the question, "How do you feel?", merely being polite, the thing to say, a kind of political correctness in our society. That has not been my judgment nor my experience.

I have viewed instead this or similar questions as expressions of genuine concern for me as a person. Below the surface there may be some hidden meanings or agenda, but the basic quest, as I witness these countless inquiries, is to merely communicate their interest and desire for my well-being.

That essentially direct inquiry, nevertheless, presents the ill person with a challenge.

One wishes to show appreciation for the others' interest or concern, but do they really want to know how I feel today, right now?

Probably not. I don't think every individual expects me to give a detailed report about my current status.

Negatively, the response might go like this: "Well, to tell you the truth, this is the week I take those darn pills and I feel lousy, got sick to my stomach yesterday and just want to sleep all the time." Positively, the response might go like this: "I am feeling better, have regained my energy, don't feel so tired, hope to run soon and to put on some lost weight."

For a public person, the sheer number of "How do you feel?" requests makes a lengthy reply like the above almost physically impossible and certainly energy draining.

As my condition has improved, I have found it necessary to develop an almost stock response.

My first desire was to receive with gratitude the presumably well-intentioned and genuinely concerned inquiry.

This is very parallel to a proper response for compliments. We can deny or deflect them, symptoms of our shaky self-image. Or we can accept and even better return them with praise, like: "I am so pleased you liked my pie. You have made my day with your compliment. Thank you for telling me how much you enjoyed it."

In that fashion, the compliment has thus been gratefully received and returned with praise.

For my situation, a simple grateful response might be expressed in this way: "I really appreciate your concern about my cancer. I am feeling better thank you."

The second desire was also to provide an honest, but brief update about my condition.

"Thanks for asking. Because of prayer and good medical treatment, I am feeling much better and the regular blood tests confirm this."

My impression is that most people are quite satisfied with such a short, but accurate answer. They seem relieved to know that I am making progress and am on the road to recovery.

14   The Road To Recovery

*T*hose struggling with any serious addictions (e.g. alcohol, drugs, sex, gambling, over or under eating) and who have undergone treatment for such diseases learn certain basic truths about their conditions.

The addiction is a disease and not their fault. Therefore, they waste their valuable energy torturing themselves with self-doubting ponderings like: "God must be punishing me," or "What a terrible person I am." There are very likely multiple causes behind the addiction, most of which are beyond the responsibility of the addicted individual.

The addiction will never go away. Treatments and twelve step programs help manage or control the disease, but never cure it. One is not a recovered, but a recovering addict. For the rest of their lives, addicted persons must continue their struggle with the addiction.

By using the means available, an addict can bring the disease under control. That means regaining order over one's life and anticipating productive, healthy and peaceful future days, providing the available means are used.

The addict needs a Higher Power beyond or outside to succeed in this lifelong struggle. For Catholics that Higher Power refers to God, the Trinity, Jesus, with the divine grace they offer to us for guidance and strength.

I found that there are parallels in my own dealings with cancer.

It is a disease and not my fault I have cancer. True, both my father and mother died of cancer, but the linkage of their disease to mine is rather tenuous. True also, I have taken pretty good care of myself physically. I have never smoked and don't drink. I exercise regularly. Except for an excess of chocolate chip cookies and probably too much red meat, my eating habits are fairly balanced.

Nevertheless, I never found myself asking, "Why me, God?" or, "How could you do this to me?" The ponderings of that young pilot about good and bad, sickness and health never entered my thinking. The issues were more: What about the future? Is this God's plan for me — some suffering for the rest of my life? How much medical care should I seek? Will I regain energy and be able to function at my former levels?

Asking God for guidance with these issues and seeking divine help for patience, courage and strength were the major thrusts of my prayer.

The disease, in my case, will never go away. It is treatable, but not curable. Some cancers, like the testicular type, can be cured, done away with, be forever gone. Others leave the patient always wondering if it will return, perhaps dreading the regular examinations and feeling relieved, especially after passing the magical five-year date, when no reoccurrence has been detected.

With Waldenstrom's disease, the hope is to cure the symptoms by reducing the cancerous cells and containing them at the normal level. But they can always emerge again to an increased degree and require new treatment.

The treatment is available, has been followed faithfully and seems to be working effectively.

If frequent recourse to God for guidance and assistance during this situation was not part of life, then I would have to question my faith, my priesthood and my pastoral ministry.

This is, then, a road to recovery, but a recovery which is limited and fragile. I am, as probably most cancer patients are, not recovered, but recovering from cancer. However, the present road is less bumpy than it was four months ago and reaching the destination of improved health, while still a limited goal, now seems more realistically and easily attainable.

A Clear Map and Detailed Triptych

At our last visit in early May, Dr. Graziano described the road we were following.

For probably a year, every six weeks I will follow the 77 pills or 11 per day for one week, then enjoy a five week breather, with blood tests every other week. During the sixth week when I come to the Regional Oncology Center for my appointment with him, there will be another blood test. This one, however, also measures the IgM count and determines the extent of the Waldenstrom's disease.

That number should gradually decrease until it is well below the safe 300 number when the treatment would be discontinued.

The red blood count or hematocrit also gauges the degree of improvement. Mine, in typical fashion for a cancer patient, had declined significantly from the normal 40 mark. At one point it stood at 26.5, low although not dangerously so, a reflection of the fatigue and sluggishness I was experiencing. The treatment should slowly increase that figure until it reaches the upper 30's. Patients who have undergone chemotherapy rarely if ever return to a 40 reading. Attaining the higher 30's, however, would justify a termination of treatments.

What then?

I would return for blood tests and a visit with him, not every two weeks, but every few months.

If the Waldenstrom's disease acts up, the numbers rise and symptoms return, we resume therapy. Should the reappearance occur after a longer interval, beyond three years, the same type of chemotherapy I have undergone would be followed. Otherwise, they must try a different medication procedure.

Dr. Graziano presented a clear map, a fairly detailed triptych of the road ahead, a methodical, hopeful and encouraging vision of what lies before me, but with some significant "ifs" or caution signs for the future.

On the Road, Again

Feeling and breathing better as well as anticipating the Memorial Day fun and fund-raising 5K or 3.2 mile race in Camillus, I arranged, as he had requested, an appointment with my friend Dr. John Fatti at his large orthopedic office.

He once again X-rayed my knees, examined the films and pronounced the 72-year-old joints as "looking better than ever." He approved the resumption of my running, but only on a gradual basis because of the five-month layoff.

Prepare carefully by heating up the knee with perhaps a hot towel. Start gradually, a half-mile today, then extend it a bit tomorrow. Don't jog more than two days at a time. Ice the knee afterwards for about five minutes, and if you feel pain in the knee, call me immediately. And some months down the road, we will get courageous and do another MRI to see what has happened with the knee.

It was the MRI in his office which had confirmed the cancer's presence and made the visit with an oncologist more urgent.

I faithfully followed his advice at the beginning of May with the race only a few weeks away. Once more a frozen pack of peas and carrots, as he suggested, proved better than a bag of ice cubes for the post-run treatment.

However, I had no idea of the surprise awaiting me when I would actively resume my jogging.

A Good Start

During the appointment with my oncologist in which Dr. Graziano laid out the map or triptych of the road ahead, he reviewed the results of my bi-weekly blood tests and the every six week test for the Waldenstrom's disease.

The news was encouraging.

The hematocrit reading had risen from 26.5 to 27.8 to 29.5. That increase did not reach the acceptable high thirty level. However, it did reflect my feeling better, disappearance of my heavy sluggishness and the return of my energy. He, after consulting with his colleagues, recommended Procrit, a widely advertised medication that is used to treat anemia. With my aversion to any other than absolutely essential drugs (the chemo pills, for example), I turned down his suggestion. Since we have made such progress in the red blood cell count, could we not wait for awhile to see if the present upward trend continues, then to judge if the current treatment seems satisfactory or not?

Dr. Graziano agreed, no doubt reluctantly, recognizing that he had a very headstrong and stubborn patient before him.

The cancer report appeared even more encouraging. The numbers had declined from 2210 to 2090 after dosage #1; from 2090 to 1610 after dosage #2.

Great news to me. The doctor concurred that something good was happening there.

It was all in all, a fine start on the final months of this road to recovery.

A Detour

The start of dosage #3 tempered that good news about improvement.

Dosage #2 had proven to be less difficult than dosage #1, but it still involved several days of struggle.

What would dosage #3 be like?

I followed the same pattern: four pills early with breakfast cereal and a little milk; three more a few hours later with more cereal and milk; four at lunch time with some food; eating very lightly at three other times during the day, with ice cream the only item which seemed appetizing.

The usual symptoms reappeared. A dread of vomiting; occasional nauseous feelings; moments of great weariness; and a need for additional naps.

I began to wonder if the light eating might be causing some of the fatigue and even the discomfort. There were no mad dashes to the bathroom and the food, however limited, reduced the nauseous feelings for a while.

On day six, I left church at noon after hearing confessions for nearly an hour and spotted the hot dog vendor in the circle in front of our church. On an impulse I purchased one (he gave me two because they were small) and ate them in the rectory. There were no bad ill effects.

That night, quite weary, hungry and feeling slightly nauseous, I drove to a pancake house and had an omelet with the accompanying pancakes. Again, no negative after effects.

Day #7 is now upon me and I still haven't decided about the possible relationship between the ill feelings and lack of adequate calories. Dosage #4 will give me another opportunity to experiment (a delightful thought).

During the midst of this challenging and difficult week, I recalled the truth "that without pain, there is no gain" and that one of the signs that the medicine is working are precisely the queasy feelings which occur. If these toxic chemo pills are in fact killing off cells, both cancerous and non-cancerous ones, then my body will react and I probably should feel, temporarily at least, "lousy." Never far from my thoughts is the realization that my own treatment causes minimal negative effects compared to the therapies for those struggling with much more aggressive cancers.

Slow, Construction Ahead

On the first day of running after my visit with the orthopedic specialist, I was starting up after a five month lay-off.

The results were devastating.

I estimated the half-mile, as he recommended, on my regular center-city route and took off for that goal. The fatigue and shortness of breath surprised me. Do you fall out of shape that fast?

The next day, I extended my trip to three quarters of a mile. Same reaction.

I took the recommended break for a day and began again, extending the run to about a mile. There was little, if any, improvement.

I finally lengthened the run to about a mile and a half.

It was a disaster. Twice or three times I had to stop running and begin walking because of weariness in my legs and shortness of breath. It brought back troublesome memories of the Memorial Day Race in Camillus a year before.

I recognized that this was in the middle of dosage #3 which certainly could have impacted my running abilities. But I had prior to the sickness run a four-mile pattern along this route with relative ease. Now I can't even make a mile without stopping!

I returned to the rectory soberly aware that I very likely would not be able to run the entire 3.2 mile route in Camillus. Nevertheless, I could still fulfill my brave, but foolish promise made several months earlier: "I intend to enter the race and finish it whether by jogging, walking, in a wheelchair or by WAVE ambulance."

Unless a miracle happens in the week before Memorial

Day, it looks like I will be running *and* walking in that race, with more of the latter than the former. A very humbling and disconcerting thought. It was indeed a major detour on this road to recovery.

But with about 400 people contributing more than $35,000 for the kids in our school to support my running on that day, the effort, despite the embarrassment, will be worthwhile.

Champion cyclist Lance Armstrong details his own bout with cancer in *It's Not About the Bike: My Journey Back to Life*. A very determined young man, he worked heroically hard to overcome obstacles and regain his ability to win a world-class bicycle race. As an older man, will I need to work equally hard to regain my own ability to jog easily four miles without stopping? Will I have that same determination?

AAA to the Rescue: Vulnerability

My four-year older brother Charles retired after more than a quarter of a century as Entertainment Editor and Film Critic for the *Los Angeles Times*. Constantly reading books and viewing films was his life work in addition to being a spouse for over 50 years, father of six and grandfather of 13.

It was, therefore, a particularly difficult day when an eye specialist declared to him: "Friend, you are legally blind." That meant no more driving; no more easy reading despite a massive machine to enlarge print; no more facile viewing of films. It also meant the impossibility of cutting your own nails or checking the menu at a restaurant.

Fortunately, he had and has his wife Peg to help with the various tasks he could no longer do by himself.

A few weeks ago Chuck and Peg traveled to New York City for a visit and an award he was to receive. I took the train there for a planned dinner together one night and a visit. We had talked on the phone often after my diagnosis, but had had no personal contact.

Soon upon arriving at my hotel room, the telephone rang. My sister-in-law called to tell me that around noon Chuck had fallen outside a restaurant, breaking hip and wrist as well as suffering an ugly forehead laceration and badly bruised eye.

An hour later in St. Clare's Hospital, I spotted this printed message over his bed: "Legally Blind." It highlighted the vulnerability that was already his and now would intensify. That would include two weeks of surgery and recuperation in a hospital and city far distant from home. Eventually, it would require an ambulance to JFK airport, special service on the American flight to Los Angeles, an ambulance to receive him there and several weeks at a Rehabilitation Center.

My brother Charles has learned about vulnerability through two major unfortunate events in his life. With no other choice, he must allow people to care for him.

Father John Finnegan had noticed the bump on his shoulder, but ignored it until that growth grew and became painful. A surgeon diagnosed and later performed rather deep surgery which left my friend in considerable pain and his arm in a sling.

The doctor advised against driving. John found he could shave and dress, but was unable to put on his socks or tie his shoes. Instead, every morning at 5:45 a very dedicated older man and parishioner would arrive at the rectory and assist him with this task. Others drove him here and there.

This very independent priest likewise learned through a difficult, although hopefully temporary, period about vulnerability, his own necessity of having others help him.

I, too, underwent a brief (six months at present) course in vulnerability. While these lessons were not as intense and essential as in my brother's case nor as awkward or painful as in Father Finnegan's situation, still, I came to realize better my need and dependence upon others.

First, my physician Dr. Gary Tyndall and his wife Ann, who has been trained as a nurse. Gary has given me very personal medical care for a dozen years, but during the months of identifying and treating the Waldenstrom's disease both have been particularly helpful. My guess is that few cancer patients have the easy access to medical advice and care during treatment that has been mine with this couple. His presentation to the parish about my condition probably highlights all that they have done for me.

Second, the medical specialists and all their colleagues. They identified the cause, outlined the cure and are implementing it.

Third, the team of the Cathedral who immediately devised ways that they could take over my responsibilities as well as shield me from phone calls and individual visitors during that early escape period.

Fourth, those people in Marcellus at St. Francis Rectory. While my time there was limited to a few weekends, they provided an essential refuge in the early period of discovery and treatment when I was at my lowest.

Fifth, that enormous support from relatives, friends, parishioners and all those people from the past and the present. Those several cartons I have of more than 1500 cards and letters symbolize this assistance and love, prayers and good wishes.

My head tells me of our need for others; this experience with cancer now has my heart believing that truth.

Lessons Learned on this Journey

During my almost yearlong journey with sickness, I have learned a number of lessons about life.

I have learned to appreciate more something I knew already — that our time on earth is limited, fleeting and unpredictable, indeed a precious gift.

I have learned that making the most of every moment is critical, lest the present now be lost through preoccupation with anticipated future events.

I have learned the sorrow and pain of experienced or expected losses — loss of energy, health, and relationships on this earth.

I have learned how blessed has been my situation with usually swift results from medical tests and how painfully anxious it must be for those who sometimes must wait at length for similar answers.

I have learned that serious illness led me to pray more faithfully and attentively, but I also learned that when I was "sick as a puppy" I became totally absorbed with myself, oblivious to others and poor at prayer.

I have learned that it helped to connect my physical challenges — a constant fatigue and shortness of breath — with Jesus' weariness on the way to Calvary and death through suffocation on the cross.

I have learned that in the early, most difficult part of my sickness, I reflected quite intensely on eternity, the life to come and reunion with people I have loved here (mother, father, stepfather).

I have learned that when you begin to feel better the intensity of prayer and those connections with the cross diminish, with one returning to life as it was.

I have learned that resolutions or conversions made during the initial dark moments tend to dissolve when your health returns or improves.

I have learned about insurance procedures, medical paperwork, oncology offices, bone marrow biopsies, blood tests, complex scans, ordinary X-rays, competent and compassionate doctors and health care workers, breathing tests, medicated inhalers, drug prescriptions and, of course, those 11 Leukeran 2MG tablets to be taken "every day for 7 days."

I have learned about just how much an incredible number of people love me and care about my well-being.

I have learned or relearned the lesson that we focus too much on the dark shadows of our lives and forget the enormous good we have done.

I have learned firsthand about the power of prayer.

I have learned, I think, how best to respond when people ask, "How do you feel?"

I have learned to expect that my health will probably improve slowly over the next months, that my anticipated future time on earth after that is uncertain, but in all probability brief (some years, not many years), and that I should live this period as well as I can knowing that sooner or later I will face God and enter eternity.

Part II
One Year Later

An Incredibly
Successful Journey

*I*t is a sunny summer Sunday, July 6, 2003, the end of a near perfect Independence Day weekend. It is also a little over a year since I stopped writing those journal-like reflections on my struggle with cancer.

Yesterday I visited at length with three couples arranging their future marriage, prepared some material for the weekend liturgies, assisted two visiting priests with the weddings of couples close to them, heard afternoon confessions from 3:45-4:45, then presided and preached at the evening Mass.

This morning I opened the church at 6:45, preached at three Masses, also presiding at one of them, celebrated two baptisms, took a short power nap and then drove the twenty or so minutes to my cottage in Skaneateles Lake for a swim prior to returning for the Sunday night 5:10 Special Young Adults Mass.

While swimming the half-mile under a clear blue sky with scattered pure white clouds, I was overwhelmed with joy and gratitude. The beautiful day and always refreshing swim were, of course, part of the reason for my uplifted spirit. Receiving word that Alba House would publish these words was another cause for the rejoicing. But most of all I felt tremendous gratitude to God for my physical well being, for the incredible restoration of full health and the remarkable effectiveness of my chemotherapy treatments.

Only twenty months ago I suffered deep fatigue, an ugly, persistent, unexplained dry cough, frequent chills and occasional night sweats. Moreover, I learned then that this rare form of blood cancer was very likely the cause of those negative symptoms.

Today, the cough is gone, the fatigue lifted, the chills are no longer, the night sweats have disappeared, and the cancer has retired at least temporarily to a dormant state.

Moreover, I feel terrific and apparently look that way to others. My energy level is what it seemed to be a decade ago; my sleep patterns, both in quality and quantity, have returned to their pre-cancer patterns; my weight has risen to what it was before the disease wreaked havoc with my body; my face is no longer gaunt and gray, but full and, in the words of a close friend, "glows with the radiance of good health."

My oncologist, Dr. Graziano, concurs that probably the cancer was present and operative several years before diagnosed. What I thought were the symptoms of being seventy, very likely were more the effects of the disease within me.

This wonderful transformation from sickness to health was not, however, an instant, miraculous cure. It came about through a yearlong treatment, a therapy planned by Dr. Graziano. His prediction was absolutely accurate. According to his plan detailed at the initial diagnosis, the slow-working treatment should within a year restore much of my former energy and free breathing. In addition, he expected that I would be able to work, even though at a lower level, while undergoing therapy.

As projected, at the one-year mark after a series of eight

dosages taken every six weeks, the cancer tests were at an acceptable level and the hematocrit reading had risen to an almost ideal mark. In addition, as I have indicated here, the visible signs of improved health reflected the positive medical testing.

I would like now to sketch this incredibly successful journey, beginning with the Memorial Day Race, 2002.

Memorial Day Race 2002

The spring 2002 newsletter for the Guardian Angel Society of Cathedral School, sent to nearly 2,000 alumni, parishioners and friends, made its annual invitation for them to support me in the 5K Memorial Day Run sponsored by the town of Camillus.

This year, however, it also described the diagnosis of my cancer and indicated that because of the disease my running had been erratic. As a result, the usual promise of an "around 30 minutes" finish probably would not be fulfilled. Nevertheless, a photo of me from the previous year's race quoted my words: "I plan to finish, whether I'm running or walking or in a wheelchair or in the back of an ambulance."

The response was enormous, the most successful in the four year history of this fundraiser for the at-risk kids in our school. No doubt some of the support could be attributed to donor awareness of my cancerous condition. Many, too, appreciated the bargain offered: For $75 we send a gift certificate, "Dinner for Two," at one of the area's finer restaurants.

Comparable contributions for 2001 and 2002 illustrate the huge response:

Year	Supporters	Gift Certificates	Donations
2001	469	273	$28,629
2002	639	391	$47,582

Concern about my cancer situation prompted some other surprising support. The Parks and Recreation Department for the town of Camillus named me as the honorary chair of the 2002 event. That meant I spoke a few words before the race began and fired the gun which started the run. Also, the first three hundred runners who registered received free "Guardian Angel Society" T-Shirts. Moreover, two dozen acquaintances decided to run with me, all wearing the same Guardian Angel shirts.

I was concerned about the race itself. I knew that I could not run the entire distance and, with so many supporters looking on, felt uncomfortable about that prospect.

However, I ran for a bit, then walked fast for awhile, ran some more, then walked, eventually arriving at the last stretch, a straight level, 1000 foot gravel path beside the Erie Canal.

At that point, a fast runner and early finisher came back and shouted to me: "Father, I already gave you $75, but if you can run the rest of the way, I will give you another $75."

Not a wise offer on his part! My competitive, greedy self took over, ignored the cancer, the fatigue, as well as everything else, and ran to the finish line.

He is now wiser and poorer.

Completion time was about 33 minutes, five minutes slower than my usual pace. But not bad for a 72 year-old and, for $47,582, certainly worth the effort.

Those Purple Pills

At the start of my treatment, I dreaded taking those tiny, purple, but potent pills daily for a week. Later, the dread softened to dislike.

When embarking every six weeks upon this seven-day chemotherapy treatment, I knew that it would quickly throw me off balance, diminish my energy and leave me feeling unwell. While I vomited only on that one occasion, the pills still caused a certain constant nausea, a queasiness. Moreover, at the end of the first day, almost on schedule, I experienced a rather severe reaction.

For example, during the first series of treatments after the Memorial Day Race, I went in the early evening for a swim. Soon after my return to shore, I began to shiver almost violently. At first I thought that it was simply a matter of becoming overchilled by the admittedly cold water. Later, as this pattern developed and became clearer, I judged that it was the instant impact of the pills.

During subsequent series of treatments, I regularly discovered and later came to expect a shutdown of my systems at the end of the initial day. That would push me to go upstairs, climb into bed, endure the chills and "shakes" for fifteen minutes or so and then fall into a deep sleep. This intense negative reaction occurred only on the first day and did not repeat itself over the next six days of pill therapy.

I also found a way to cope with the nausea. When those feelings appeared every few hours, I would forget the repugnance I had for food, go to the kitchen and eat a cracker or a cookie. That temporarily quieted the queasiness.

It seemed like the pills were working furiously within my

stomach and, without food there, created the nausea. The slight intake of some nourishment appeared to eliminate that queasiness without minimizing the pills' effectiveness.

We know the theory that radiation or chemotherapy destroys the bad cells, but also some good ones. It is not surprising then, that we suffer unpleasantries during the treatment periods.

While I detested and disliked those purple pills and their effects, my treatment was minimal compared to the therapy many must suffer with cancer.

A close friend, to illustrate, endured deep surgery for the removal of a 3" by 1" cancerous growth on his shoulder, followed by surgical removal of the lymph nodes to ensure no cancer remained. This was followed by Interferon, an extremely strong anti-cancer drug. My friend reacted so violently to the medication that they had to discontinue his therapy and merely hope that his cancer will never return.

While my treatment was actually easy in comparison to many of the other therapies, those little pills were nevertheless most effective as you can see from the discussion and data which follows.

Proof of Progress

There is usually, although not always, a correlation between medical tests and feeling better (or worse). That certainly did occur in my case.

As I began to feel better, the bad numbers gradually declined. From a high of 2210, the IgM count reached a low of 120, an acceptable and normal level. Conversely, as my energy returned, the hematocrit level rose, from the lowest level of 26.5 to the high of 40.1. A reading much below 26.5 will often require a blood transfusion; a 40 reading is almost ideal for a 73-year-old man.

The chart below documents these gradual and also encouraging increments.

Laboratory Results

	1/22/02	3/28/02	5/09/02	6/20/02	8/13/02	9/24/02	11/12/02	2/6/03	3/27/03	5/19/03
Hct	31.6	27.8	29.5	28.5	32.9	32.9	35.7	37.8	38.9	40.1
IgM	2210	2090	1610	1220	1420	1170	832	252	182	130

*NOTE: **Normal values for adult Hct is 41-53.**
Normal values for the Igm is 60-263 mg/dl.

Dr. Tyndall who prepared this chart and the graph below explains in greater detail the meaning of these numbers:

The initial blood studies were done on 1/22/02, prior to the start of chemotherapy. The tests on 3/28/02 were done after his first course of chemotherapy. As you can see from the chart he had a steady and progressive fall in his serum IgM. This is a reflection of the success of his chemotherapy in eradicating the cancer cells producing this substance in excess. In concert with the fall of his IgM, the Hematocrit (Hct), commonly known as your blood count began to rise and has returned to an almost normal level as of 5/19/03. This reflects the ability of his bone marrow to resume production of normal cells once the marrow was no longer over-whelmed by the abnormal cancer cells.

Laboratory Results

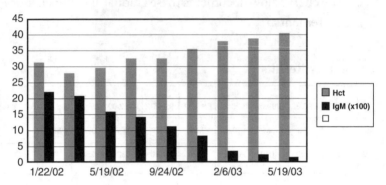

On July 17, 2003, I had, at Dr. John Fatti's suggestion, an MRI on my knee similar to the earlier one which had re-vealed the presence of the cancer. The new images were, in his words, "incredible, totally different, almost miraculous, with-out a sign of cancer."

Good Side Effects

We have countless human experiences in which something good emerges from something bad, when light emerges in the midst of darkness, when negative developments lead surpris-ingly to positive effects.

The Bible provides a biblical and theological basis for this phenomenon. Paul writing to the Christians at Rome reminded them of that truth in these words: "We know that all things work for good for those who love God..." (Romans 8:28).

As I interpret his teaching, God leaves human beings free to make choices, right and wrong ones. But when situations develop, particularly negative developments, the loving Creator somehow brings positive results out of those circumstances.

Two current incidents in my life illustrate this notion.

Joan and Tom were scheduled to be married at the Cathedral three months after I was diagnosed with cancer. As a result, they became two of the first persons to learn of my situation and immediately wondered whether I would be able to perform the ceremony. I was and did.

However, a week after that quite tearful session discussing the wedding possibilities, this wonderful couple left a gift for me: a copy of *Theodore Rex*, an account of Teddy Roosevelt's presidency. They thought that during my treatment period I might have more quiet moments for reading than usual.

I have read a good bit during my adult life and through the priesthood of 47 years. But except for novels during vacation, the fare has been almost entirely spiritual or theological books — works helpful to my prayer life or pastoral work. Seldom, however, have I gotten into history.

This gift and a shift in my daily pattern changed that. Now, prior to retiring, I often read for about a half hour some historical or current event volume. The experience has been enjoyable, enriching and useful.

When I look at the stack of such books finished over the past two years, it reminds me of the truth that one who reads consistently, even if for a few moments each day, will cover much material.

My nephew Chuck and his wife Bonnie two weeks ago suffered the tragedy parents of a baby consciously or unconsciously fear. Emily Catherine, eight months old, their only child, was placed in her crib for an afternoon nap. Seemingly a perfectly healthy infant, she just stopped breathing.

There followed an instant call to 911, CPR, the ambulance rush to University Hospital's Pediatric Emergency Unit, expert health care personnel furiously working on the baby — all to no avail.

That night I sat beside the numb, disbelieving, crushed parents for two hours. I grieved with them and eventually helped this couple make a few necessary decisions — funeral director, burial plot, possible services. We had several other moments together in the days ahead, including the funeral and my taking them to dinner a week later so they could visit about coping with their loss.

There were many positive side effects to this terribly dark event for all involved, including the parents. For me, it was feeling a great closeness to my nephew and his spouse, a new and tighter bond that presumably will remain forever.

Puerto Rico and Camillus Revisited

What a difference one year makes!

In February of 2002, during a few days at Puerto Rico, I received a phone call confirming my cancer, spent many sad, tearful moments by a pool pondering the uncertain future, and could barely carry on a conversation at dinner because of the incessant cough.

Chills and night sweats made sleep fitful and hardly refreshing. Not able to run or jog at all, my exercise was limited to a short walk in the nearby park.

One year later, February 2003, during another several days at Puerto Rico, I was no longer receiving chemotherapy, the negative symptoms had all disappeared and I sat by the pool overwhelmed with gratitude for the remarkable restoration of my health.

This recovery was probably dramatized on the first day there when I, with relative ease, resumed my usual five mile run from the hotel along the ocean to Old San Juan, and back.

On Memorial Day, 2002, described earlier in this chapter, I completed the 5K Camillus Race, but in limited fashion. While vastly improved and on the road to recovery, I still could only run a bit, then walk, run again, then walk.

On Memorial Day, 2003, now fully recovered and re-energized, I had complete confidence that I could run the 3.2 miles without stopping.

I did, a little slower than my usual healthy pace, in 30:30 minutes, but under extremely restrictive weather conditions. A pouring rain left all the runners soaked through to the skin and the last part of the journey, that 1,000 foot gravel path, filled with puddles of water.

Nevertheless, I finished #1 in my category of those 70 or over. Although most likely I was the only one in that division, I still received as my prize a pair of running socks and two $1.00 gift certificates for McDonalds.

And I raised $38,824 for the kids at our school.

Several Serious Scares and Divine Nudges

Persons who have recovered from malfunctioning heart conditions or whose cancers are in remission often become very sensitive to any symptoms which may indicate a reoccurrence of those health problems. I certainly fit into that category. Over a relatively short period after completing my chemotherapy, I experienced several serious medical scares and, with them, what I have come to term gentle divine nudges.

The first began early in 2003. I had felt, but could not see, a sore spot on the crown of my head. My barber said it looked like a sort of pimple. My medical friends concurred, thought it showed signs of a minor infection and recommended some standard at home procedures to rectify the problem.

Unfortunately, those measures failed to correct the situation; that bump appeared to grow and the soreness intensified.

Here is where the first divine nudge occurred. After several weeks, I felt an inclination to check this out with my dermatologist, but hesitated to do so lest my personal physician friend be offended. Strangely, without a word from me, he now urged I do just that.

The skin specialist examined my spot, judged it could be cancerous and obtained through biopsy a sample for laboratory study.

A few days later he called, informed me that it indeed was a squamous cell carcinoma, needed removal and, because of its location, recommended a plastic surgeon.

The surgeon subsequently reassured me that while the cancerous growth needed to be excised, there was little danger of its spreading beyond the scalp area. Busy schedules, his and mine, meant an almost month delay before the operation could be performed.

Shortly thereafter, I felt another of those divine nudges, an impulse leading me to call the surgeon's receptionist, asking to be placed on the cancellation list for a possible earlier opening. One surfaced within a few days.

The operation was relatively simple, although I had some fears about it beforehand. The gentle and obviously skilled surgeon numbed my scalp, made a two-inch incision, removed the cancerous section and a bit of surrounding tissue for laboratory examination, sutured the wound and electrically cauterized the flow of blood.

During that last part of the surgery, I suddenly felt a sharp shock. Lying by my side on the operating table, I had inadvertently placed a hand on the metal rod at the edge of the table. Noting my reaction, the doctor apologized, "Oh, I forgot to tell you that it would be best not to touch the metal while I am doing this."

Following surgery, the doctor observed that the cancer was more aggressive than he had thought and that I had wisely come earlier for its removal.

For a week, I was to treat the wound and wear a bandage

patch on the top of my head. I tried once at the beginning with mirrors to do this myself, only to be told later by my medical friends that the bandage was an inch away from the cut. They graciously performed the needed care after that.

Another nudge happened during the healing period.

Several "street" people spend time in the park-like circle before our Cathedral. One of them sits or lies on the sidewalk, sometimes sleeping overnight out in the open.

Blessed with a brilliant mind, the man is clear, coherent and quite spiritual when in a good mood. But when a dark period overtakes him, he becomes incoherent, vile and even violent. He thus poses an ongoing challenge for us.

One afternoon I walked by him as he sat on the sidewalk feeding pigeons. He called out to me, but I pretended not to hear the man, wishing to avoid another unpleasant encounter.

He called again. This time one of those divine nudges moved me to acknowledge his greeting.

"What's that patch on your head?" he asked.

"I have a skin cancer which was surgically removed."

He responded, to my surprise, with genuine concern, "I hope it turns out all right for you."

During my return and final visit the surgeon reported that all the surrounding edges of the removed material were cancer free. Moreover, he performed his task with such skill that today there is barely a trace of the two-inch incision.

The second scare surfaced shortly thereafter.

For a few weeks I had experienced a slight soreness over

my left breast. One night, while showering, I realized that the flesh surrounding the nipple was hard and swollen.

Since I soon had a regularly scheduled appointment with my oncologist, I decided to wait until then for his examination of this new development. But then another of those nudges took over.

I mentioned it to my nurse friend who immediately said her physician husband should examine the swelling that night. He did, was puzzled by the symptoms, and arranged for me to visit a general surgeon within the next few days.

During that appointment this kind and highly regarded doctor looked at and felt my breast, then gave his analysis.

"This is probably something called gynecomastia, rare and found usually in adolescent boys and older men. We do not know what causes the growth nor can much be done about it. It is 97% certain that you have this; there is a 3% chance it could be cancer, although I doubt that based on my examination. If cancerous, the breast must be removed; otherwise, we do nothing. A biopsy is the only way to determine whether we are looking at cancer or the other development. I have two appointments ahead of me. If you care to wait, we can do the surgery this afternoon."

The wait lasted for nearly an hour. While somewhat, but not overly anxious, I began walking around the operating table. Knowing that the biopsy would be unpleasant, although not exceedingly so, I thought about offering to God the worry and discomfort for several persons in serious need. During this circular journey, I brought to mind a half-dozen such people, asking the Lord to look upon my ordeal and bless them.

Of my three biopsies — the bone marrow, the scalp and now the breast — this was the most difficult.

At one point the surgeon asked, "Are you all right? You look pale."

I replied, "Yes. Probably just scared and nervous."

Afterwards he said, "Call me in two days and we will have the results."

Those were very, very anxious days. I imagined the worst case scenario, of course: cancer, breast removal, radiation, and chemotherapy. The other inevitable question arose: If it is cancer, do I undergo such treatment?

I called as requested, but the receptionist said the results would not be available for four days instead of the two indicated. The surgeon must have then intervened, because later in the afternoon he telephoned and announced, to my great relief, that the growth was not cancerous, but of the other kind.

Today I have a still slightly swollen and hardened left breast with a barely distinguishable scar, but no cancer.

With this scare over, I next visited my dentist for a semi-annual checkup. All seemed well until the hygienist began mumbling to herself and kept exploring the left inside of my mouth.

When my dentist stopped in, he examined a red spot that had troubled her, held a mirror before me, pointed out the small circular redness, and declared: "With your history of cancer, I want you to see Dr. Paul Fallon, the oral surgeon, and have him check this spot. It is asymmetrical and changes color when I move it around."

It was disheartening news. I immediately had images of complex jaw surgery with subsequent intense therapy and asked myself again: Would I go through this type of aggressive, radical treatment should the spot be cancerous?

The very next day, I was sitting in Dr. Fallon's chair. The oral surgeon looked and saw nothing serious, simply some normal tissue discoloration. He asked his son, also an oral surgeon, to examine the spot. The younger physician agreed with his father and described the phenomenon as a hemangioma. However, he suggested I come back for a check-up one month later.

On that return visit, I sat in the waiting room with a husband and wife plus three teenagers, two of whom were apparently facing oral surgery. As the young people were checking in the receptionist asked: "You are the ones going to sleep, right?"

In a few minutes, a nurse called in the married couple, the husband reappearing shortly thereafter. He said, with an impish smile, "You should see that needle!" The two teenagers about to be put to sleep for surgery practically died on the spot.

My own session lasted less than two minutes. A check of the area; same diagnosis; no need to return. The dentist, he said, will keep abreast of the situation with his regular examinations.

The fourth and final scare was more of a familiar and wearisome burden than a scare.

It was familiar, because over the past two decades I have undergone treatment for skin cancers on many occasions.

It was wearisome, because in only a few months time I had visited a plastic surgeon, a general surgeon, an oral surgeon and now, finally, the dermatologist who initiated these events.

The fact is that I have been paying the price for those hours of unprotected swimming in the sun as a young boy and a not so young adult. That dermatologist has regularly burned, scraped and excised various developing skin cancers from my face, scalp and back. This particular appointment would not differ from previous ones.

After examining my body literally from top to bottom for signs of actual or potential skin cancer, he located nine spots needing attention.

In my medical history with him, that was a record for a single visit. There were four on the right side of my face, two on the left including a growth near my eye, and three on the crown of my head.

Armed with a cotton-tipped wooden applicator in one hand and his seemingly always present mug of misting liquid nitrogen in the other, he swiftly burned away the dangerous looking areas. ("Oh! This probably stings more on the top of your head because the scalp is very sensitive.")

I was then given the standard follow-up treatment instruction sheet. ("Clean the site twice a day with alcohol. You can shower or get the locations wet. It will blister and heal in 1-2 weeks.") He added another step: "Ice-pack the site near your eye twice a day for three minutes. Otherwise, the treated area will swell and cause a closed, blackened eye." Finally, the dermatologist told me to make an appointment with the receptionist for nine months later.

Fortunately, in my case, these treated sites heal very swiftly and within several days the scars were hardly noticeable.

I must thank the dentist who twenty years ago noted suspicious signs on my face and suggested a visit to this dermatologist. If I had not followed his recommendations then, my situation now would likely be quite different, probably ugly and perhaps fatal.

It was a few months of serious scares. Fortunately, the conditions were either not serious, or, with relative ease, quite treatable. In addition, I experienced those divine nudges and gained spiritual insights from them.

Looking Back
and Ahead

On a splendid August weekday in 2002, I made my annual trip north for a visit with friends Dr. Gary and Ann Tyndall at their summer home by the St. Lawrence River in Morristown, New York.

A beautiful sky and lush green foliage made the two-hour drive a joy in itself. Upon arrival, I followed what has become a standard routine: lunch, a nap for me, the three of us running at an easy pace for a few miles, a dip in the river, then dinner at an elegant restaurant in Alexandria Bay celebrating their wedding anniversary.

During the night drive back to Syracuse, I felt very grateful for a most pleasant day away from work and with close friends.

But there were three glitches in the otherwise perfect visit: I was still on chemotherapy; I had to fight drowsiness during the last part of the journey north; my nap was in reality an hour-long deep sleep.

I am writing this third and final chapter after having made, yesterday, the Summer 2003 trip north to spend a day with those friends. The scenario was identical in almost every respect from the previous year. However, there were three differences:

my chemotherapy, at least temporarily, has been discontinued; I felt no drowsiness driving; a mere ten-minute nap totally refreshed me.

As I look back over the past two years of symptoms, diagnosis and treatment, these specific examples above illustrate why gratitude is the dominant theme in my reflections.

Looking Back with Gratitude

I am grateful most of all to *God* for such an incredibly successful medical journey and this remarkable restoration of my health.

God is the giver of every gift from above, a God who helps and heals, a God, however, who seeks our loving gratitude for these blessings.

Christian, Jewish and Muslim religious traditions echo those concepts. Each in different ways acknowledge the divine origin of everything and the consequent human responsibility to give thanks to God both individually and together with others.

My quiet reflective prayer every morning tends to be filled with these sentiments of gratitude as I ponder this or that health blessing. Moreover, when I fulfill our Catholic worship, especially the Mass and the Liturgy of the Hours, the rituals frequently contain texts which speak about giving thanks.

Today, for example, is the feast of Our Lady of Mount Carmel. The Greek word for Mass, Eucharist, itself means to give thanks. The preface for this feast contains the phrase: "We do well always and everywhere to give you thanks." An introductory dialogue to that preface, standard for all prefaces, includes this invitation and response:

Priest: "Let us give thanks to the Lord our God."

People: "It is right to give him thanks and praise."

During the words of institution, the Mass formula reminds us that at the Last Supper, Jesus "gave thanks." Finally, the psalm response for this feast of Our Lady of Mount Carmel uses a verse from St. Luke's Gospel in which Mary, the mother of Jesus, gratefully praises God with these words: "The Almighty has done great things for me, and holy in his name" (Luke 1:49).

Those public expressions of gratitude now have fresh and deeper meaning for me.

I am also grateful to God for those lessons about life learned through this struggle. I listed them in Chapter 14 of Part I and try to make these truths part of my daily living.

God does heal, but usually uses human instruments to achieve that purpose. Looking back has also, therefore, renewed my gratitude for those *many supportive people* who surrounded me with love, prayers and even practical assistance during the treatment period.

From get-well cards to history books, from a welcoming rectory to coverage of the Cathedral, from spoken words of concern to weekend prayers for me at parishes, the outpouring of love has been enormous.

Now that my health has returned to normal, I am suddenly taken aback by the question: "How are you feeling?"

Then I realize that since there has been no public announcement of my recovery, the inquirer is still praying for me, without any realization of my improved condition. I fumble for an answer and need to develop a sincere, but standard response like this: "Thank you for your concern and prayers. With God's help, great medical care and much love, I am actually feeling very fine, 100%, back to my good health of six years ago."

I am also, of course, deeply grateful to the many *health care professionals* who made my struggle easier and successful.

To Doctor Gary Tyndall, whose contact with other physicians surely gave me almost immediate access to them and special attention starting with the oncologist and continuing through those several serious scares. To his wife and trained nurse Ann who drove me home from the Regional Oncology Center (ROC) when I was still giddy from the Demerol, dressed the scalp incision which I could not see and helped in other ways too numerous to count.

To Doctor John Fatti who arranged the knee X-rays and MRI, then sat before me with great empathy as I faced the fact that the presence of cancer had been confirmed by those tests.

To oncologist Doctor Steven Graziano who for two years has been always gentle and competent, while ready with a clear plan of treatment and uncanny in his time prediction of successful results. And to his team members at ROC, including the laboratory technicians who regularly gave me, as soon as possible, printouts of the blood test numbers during my anxious wait for an improvement in hematocrit scores.

To Doctor Robert Lenox, that lung specialist who provided me with the first good news during a dark time and to the hospital's respiratory staff in their cramped testing space who measured my lung capacity, finding it far below normal.

To those doctors and dentists, with their supporting colleagues, who so swiftly and expertly diagnosed and/or treated the several serious scares described in chapter two of this part.

I sent to all of those offices a can or two of the world's greatest peanuts as an expression of my gratitude. Those few words are an added attempt to express my appreciation.

Looking Ahead with Trust

As I look ahead in my 73rd year, feeling exceptionally well, I do so with trust, with a sense of abandonment to God, surrendering to whatever the future may hold. "Letting go," was a phrase, as we noted earlier, which emerged for the late Joseph Cardinal Bernardin during struggles with three heavy burdens at the end of his life, including a fatal cancer. If we "let go," he wrote, "if we place ourselves totally in the hands of the Lord, the good will prevail."

That trust, abandonment and "letting go" applies to three current aspects of my life.

The Disease. I know Waldenstrom's disease is incurable and supposedly will rise at some point from the normal to a destructive level. Even though my most recent tests show acceptable readings and even a continued decline in the cancer's presence, studies indicate the median duration of survival is 5.4 years, with 20% of patients living as long as 10 years. However, one person told me after a meeting that her husband had this disease at 67 and lived to 93!

So, right now, I am at peace, simply "letting go" of worry about the future of this cancer.

My Age. I am unusually healthy, active and energetic for a man in his 70's. But sooner, rather than later, this will certainly change. However, for the moment, staying the course means beginning each morning with prayerful gratitude, living fully the hours which follow and, again, letting go of concern about an ultimate decline in my health.

Retirement. Friends and others frequently ask, "Will you retire?" or "Are you thinking about retirement?" or "When will you retire?"

My response is always the same: it depends upon my physical, emotional and mental health. When my health deteriorates and impedes my work or burdens parishioners, then it will be time. Or when I no longer have the vision or energy to lead the Cathedral and our team forward, then it will be time.

Now, however, especially with the shortage of priests and the condition of the Church in America, does not seem to be the time.

Unfortunately, as older persons we tend not to recognize the decline in health or the stagnation of enthusiasm. For that reason, I have asked close friends to tell me, out of their love, when that condition has arrived and it is finally the time to retire.

Until then, I am quite content to let go and to trust, to abandon and to surrender.

From Time to Eternity and Back

This account began at a surprise party on my 70th birthday accompanied by a few subsequent reflections on that particular time in my life and some questions about the decade ahead.

I certainly had no inkling then that the next three years would involve a serious struggle with cancer.

During those difficult early months of treatment, I had a brush with eternity and reflected with some intensity about life after death.

Now I am back in time, but with a different focus or emphasis: seeking to live gratefully, productively and fully the present moment in time, but with greater awareness of the world to come.

Cardinal Bernardin concluded his chapter on "Letting Go" in this way: These "are simply reflections from my heart to yours. I hope they will be of help to you in your own life so you too can enjoy the deep inner peace — God's wonderful gift to me — that I now embrace as I stand on the threshold of eternal life."

I would like to make his sentiments my own.

Acknowledgments

I had no idea at my ordination that after nearly a half-century in the priesthood I would have published over 50 works with more than 20 million copies in circulation, authored a weekly national column for 17 years, and traveled about two million miles lecturing here and abroad on pastoral topics.

However, in those early creative days I soon learned a truth about myself. When touched deeply by an experience, I invariably processed the personal event through writing. The situation moving me might be a film or a novel, a beautiful nature scene or a fine musical performance, a personal exchange or a pastoral encounter.

This three year struggle with cancer was, of course, probably the most traumatic event in my life. Writing about it, therefore, simply followed my customary pattern. Nevertheless, transferring these experiences immediately to paper when they happened, as I did in Part I, no doubt also became a catharsis for me.

Several local people urged me to have my recollections published. These included members of the Cathedral team, Danielle Cummings, the Communication Director for the Diocese of Syracuse, and Richard Case, an at large columnist for our daily newspaper, the *Post-Standard*.

All of us, consequently, were delighted when Father Edmund C. Lane, S.S.P., of Alba House on Staten Island accepted the manuscript (Part I) and expressed his desire to publish the book as soon as possible. I then quickly developed Part II as an addition to the original text.

I have expressed my gratitude to the health care personnel and named a few doctors within the text itself. Here I wish to acknowledge with deep appreciation all those doctors and dentists who were so good to me: Doctors R.J. Dietz, Paul Fallon, Timothy Fallon, John Fatti, Stephen Graziano, Robert Lenox, Jon Lochner, John Sullivan, Mohammed Tabaie, David Tyler and Gary Tyndall.

Three persons with wisdom and patience transferred my handwritten pages first to the computer and then on to the diskette: Maureen Quirk, Ann Tyndall and Julie Tyndall. They also contributed helpful comments and insights as did several early readers of the Part I draft. I am very grateful to all of them.

I cited and quoted a few valuable volumes in the course of my book. They are listed here for easy reference in the order as they appear in my text:

The Gift of Peace. Joseph Cardinal Bernardin (Chicago and New York: Loyola Press and Doubleday, 1997-8). Part I:8; Part II:17.

Pastoral Care of the Sick. (New York: Catholic Book Publishing Company, 1983). Part I:8.

Life After Life. Raymond Moody (New York: Bantam Books, 1975). Part I:9.

When the Dying Speak. Ron Wooten Green (Chicago: Loyola Press, 2001). Part I:9.

Acknowledgments

Charming Billy. Alice McDermott (New York: Dell Publishing, 1999). Part I:9.

It's Not About the Bike. Lance Armstrong (New York: Berkley Books, 2001). Part I:14.

For privacy's sake I did not identify those individuals whose loving and supportive comments occur in Part I, 11-12. I deeply appreciated their notes then and their appearance now in this book. I likewise want to express my gratitude to friends, Sister Charla Commins, C.S.J. and Ms. Patricia Livingston Gordon whose insights are included within the volume.

If I have neglected to credit any contributor, please contact me and I will make every effort to correct that in the future.

Finally, Ann and Gary Tyndall, as the book demonstrates, have been by my side from the start and at every moment of this struggle. I cannot thank them enough for their presence, love and assistance.

Father Joseph M. Champlin
Rector, Cathedral of the Immaculate Conception
Syracuse, New York
Summer, 2003